WALL PILATES

FOR
SENIORS

INCLUDES CHAIR EXERCISES TOO!

77 Illustrated, low-impact exercises in 2 customizable routines, to help you lose weight, improve your mobility and flexibility, and to increase your energy and independence

IVY THOMAS

BUT FIRST, A FEW QUOTES ABOUT AGING...

"You can't help getting older, but you don't have to get old."

~George Burns

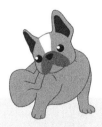

"Aging is not lost youth, but a new stage of opportunity and strength."

~Betty Friedan

"Every moment of our life can be the beginning of great things."

~Joseph Pilates

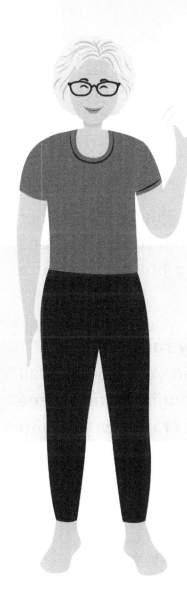

"Your 40s are good. Your 50s are great. Your 60s are fab. And 70 is f*@king awesome!"

~Helen Mirren

Now on to some quick start questions you might have...

QUICK START FAQ

Will Wall Pilates really work?

Wall Pilates is deceptively simple-looking, but the exercises are very effective because they target specific muscles in an isolated, yet supportive way. You'll read more about that in Chapter 1 and you'll experience it as you practice your routine.

Does the book only have Wall Pilates?

This book focuses on Wall Pilates, but it also utilizes Chair Pilates as another supportive way to exercise. After the Pilates routines, there are also sections on nutrition, as well as mental and social wellness, for a holistic look at a healthy, joyful lifestyle.

Are there any prerequisites before starting the 28-day routine?

No, there are no prerequisites you need before you begin your 28-day Wall Pilates journey, but I highly recommend that you go through the first three short chapters before you do. The goal of this book is to empower you with knowledge and set you up for long-term success.

How much activity do I actually need?

Older adults 65 and up need:

- **150 minutes of moderate or vigorous-intensity activity weekly.**
- **strength training twice per week.**
- **activities that will improve balance.**

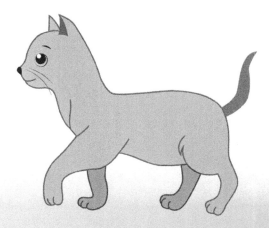

How does this tie into Wall Pilates?

Wall Pilates is a mix of balance and strength, so when you implement Wall Pilates into your routine and get up to three times a week, you will check the balance and strength activities off your weekly activity list.

Can I combine Wall Pilates with other fitness activities?

As you get more flexible, mobile and stronger from practicing Wall Pilates, you should add in activities that will satisfy your body's moderate to vigorous cardio needs. This can come from:

- **five 30-minute walks (moderate intensity) or two 75-minute hikes or jogs (vigorous-intensity), or a mix of the two**
- **other leisure activities, such as golfing, bowling or pickleball**
- **swimming or participating in aqua fitness classes**
- **If you already do some of the above activities, or something comparable, incorporating Wall Pilates will round out your fitness routine properly. Not only that, it will improve your ability to perform your current cardio at a more effective level.**

How often should I practice Wall Pilates to see noticeable improvements?

To see the benefits and improvements from practicing Wall Pilates, you should practice at least 3 times a week for 30 to 45 minutes. However, listen to your body and don't push it too aggressively to get up to that amount. Be mindful as you go, and you'll get there for sure!

ABOUT THE AUTHOR

Meet Ivy Thomas, a vibrant woman whose journey into the world of fitness and wellness launched with a significant personal milestone: a total knee replacement at the age of 53. Determined to regain her strength and vitality, Ivy tried various forms of exercise until she came across Wall Pilates—a revelation that would transform her life. Inspired by its supportive approach and its emphasis on the power of small movements, Ivy embraced Wall Pilates wholeheartedly, experiencing firsthand its remarkable effects on her body. As she witnessed her own physical rejuvenation and newfound agility, Ivy became passionate about sharing this empowering practice with others, particularly those navigating the challenges of rehabilitation and aging. With her own parents in their eighties, Ivy understands firsthand the importance of maintaining mobility and vitality as we age. Through her writing, Ivy hopes to inspire others to discover the transformative potential of Wall Pilates, proving that age is no barrier to living a vibrant and fulfilling life.

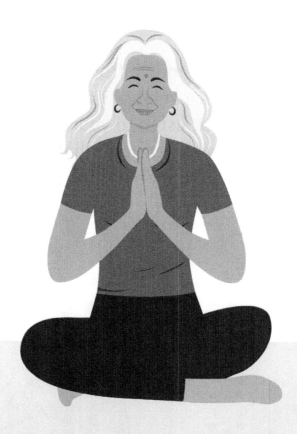

TABLE OF CONTENTS

JOIN THE **FOREVER FIT FOLKS** CONTENT TEAM!

At Forever Fit Folks, we want to tailor our content to the needs of our readers, like you! Join our early feedback and review team so that we can get your thoughts about what you'd like to see next!

Scan the QR code!

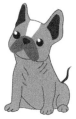

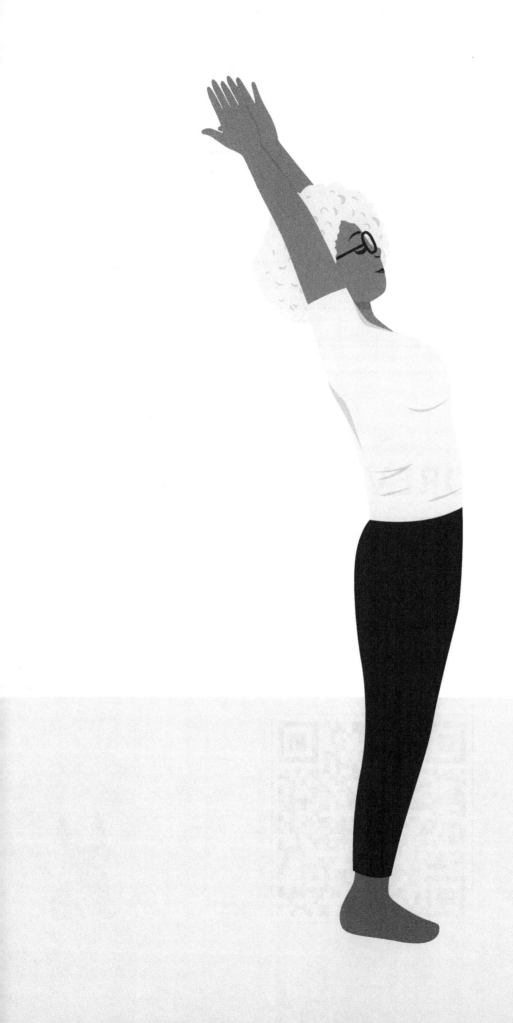

INTRODUCTION

I don't know about you, but I want to feel fabulous and awesome about my life!

Being vibrant for life is not only important, it's completely achievable. Being in a Senior age bracket doesn't have to signal slowing down or becoming dependent on others. It simply means that we need to practice fitness and self-care in a way that supports our specific fitness level and goals.

The more you move, the better your joints are lubricated. The better your joints, flexibility and balance are, the more you can do activities that build muscle and strength. The stronger you are, the better you feel and can pursue doing anything you want. Your end goal can be an active one such as biking, hiking and playing racket sports, or it can be as fundamental as walking up and down stairs without pain, improving your circulation and being able to do some cardio to take care of your heart and lungs.

It's all about how we see our lifelong health and how we approach it. Aging is a fact of life, but *how* we age is a culmination of what we do every day, starting with the small steps we take today. Everything we do from today onwards shapes who we'll be and how we'll be in 6 months, a year, in 3 years, and so on. But it's largely in our control, and that's a powerful thing to truly understand.

While this book has been written with Senior fitness in mind, Wall Pilates is for anyone. It's a targeted, practical exercise method that challenges your muscles with small movements in a low-impact, yet powerful way. You'll be surprised at how easy and effective small, consistent exercise can be to build muscle, improve range of motion, increase your flexibility, your balance, help you lose weight and maintain or increase your independence.

Throughout *Wall Pilates for Seniors*, you will be given a step-by-step approach to improving your overall health. These exercises have been tailored to target specific muscles, joints and pain relief, incorporating both the wall and a chair for support, and there's a customizable 28-day routine to follow for different levels of ability as you go. In addition, this book will teach you how to integrate other physical, mindful and emotional activities for a holistic approach to wellness that really supercharges your quality of life!

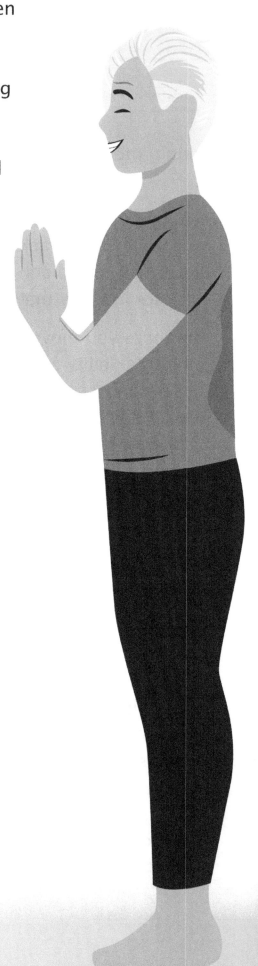

CHAPTER 1:

WHAT THE HECK ARE WALL PILATES AND HOW WILL THEY HELP ME?

Wall Pilates is a modification of traditional Pilates with many applications, but to know the true benefits of it, you'll need to have a basic understanding of what Pilates is and the power of it.

An Introduction to Pilates

In essence, Pilates is a series of small targeted muscle exercises, combined with resistance that develops one's lean muscle mass, strength, flexibility and balance.

Joseph Pilates created the method in 1883 by rigging the springs on hospital beds so bedridden soldiers could use the power of resistance to exercise. This was the start of Pilates and its reformer systems.

Joseph later moved to New York and opened up a fitness studio and by the late 1960s, Pilates was becoming popular worldwide. Because Pilates has such great results, this form of exercise has remained a popular option for all ages.

What Is the Difference Between Pilates and Wall Pilates?

In the traditional form of Pilates, the practice is mainly done on a mat or with a Pilates reformer machine.

Wall Pilates takes the exercises you would otherwise do on the floor or with a reformer, and puts them against the wall or on a chair to add stability, support and resistance. In Wall Pilates, you'll have less stress or pressure on your spine, knees, hips and joints, making it an ideal workout for many, especially those looking for a low-intensity activity that works. It's also an excellent option for anyone who has limited mobility and finds getting up and down from the floor more difficult.

The Benefits of Wall Pilates for Seniors

Improved Balance and Stability

Wall Pilates increases core strength. Also, the mind-body connection that Pilates promotes helps to increase our body's ability to sense its surroundings. Together, these improve our balance.

Improved Flexibility and Mobility

Wall Pilates exercises lubricate our joints and stretch our muscles, developing a greater range of motion and flexibility.

Improved Posture

Using the wall as support during Pilates improves the alignment of our spine, and will leave you standing taller, with less shoulder or neck tension.

Improved Circulation

With the deep breathing component of Wall Pilates, you improve your overall circulation, allowing your organs to continue functioning well and reducing the risk of heart disease or stroke.

Full-Body Conditioning

Wall Pilates exercises activate several muscle groups at the same time. Each exercise targets your core, arms, legs, and glutes in small ways simultaneously.

Gentle on Joints and Reduces Inflammation

The low impact approach that Wall Pilates brings to resistance training is gentle and supportive on your joints.

Supports and Increases Rehabilitation

Pilates has been used for years to help overcome injuries. Using a wall and chair for support is even more helpful in a rehabilitation plan for back, knee and shoulder pain.

Stress Relief and Relaxation

The inward focus that Wall Pilates promotes with its breathing and the mind-body connection is an excellent way to boost your mood and energy.

Easy Access

Wall Pilates is available to everyone of all levels and abilities. Everyone has a wall in their house so the only extra pieces of equipment you will need are a mat and a chair and potentially a stability wall or some light weights.

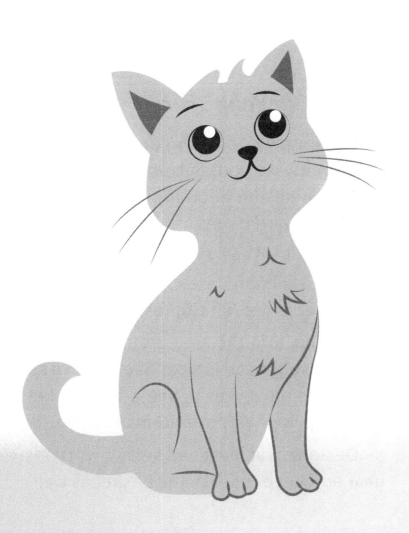

CHAPTER 2:

SETTING UP AT HOME SO YOU CAN DO IT ANYTIME!

Take a few minutes now to design your exercise routine for success. You'll want a dedicated space of your own and to create a motivating atmosphere for yourself.

Creating a Comfortable Exercise Environment

With Wall Pilates, you only need a space where you can roll out **a yoga mat**, ideally near the corner of two **sturdy walls**, that you have consistent access to. You'll also need a sturdy chair and likely a stability ball hand, and that's fundamentally it!

Tips to Enhancing Your Space

Next is the fun part - creating an atmosphere that will motivate you! Set up the space to feel functional and good for you. You want to look forward to getting into your space and taking care of your body.

· Natural light is best, or a space with brighter white light bulbs.

· Make sure the area around you and above your head is clear of obstacles so you can move freely, and add a basket to keep your workout items handy.

· Designate at least two sets of workout gear and keep those in the basket as well.

You should wear non-slip workout socks or simply be in your bare feet when exercising.

· Always have water available so you can stay hydrated when exercising. Another item for the basket is a water bottle that makes you happy.

· Have a good temperature in the room. You don't want to feel heated or too cold.

· Ideally (but not required), you'd have a mirror installed opposite you, so that you're able to see what you're doing and can adjust your body as needed.

· Cheer up the space with a plant, a motivating photo of a result you're wanting to achieve, etc.

· Have a mobile speaker you can play music on, or have your phone nearby with a playlist that you enjoy.

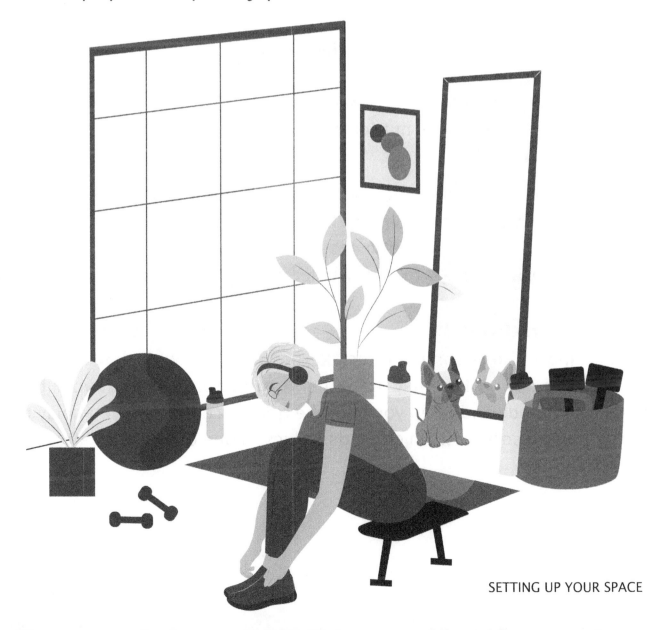

CHAPTER 3:

STARTING RIGHT - WARMING UP, BREATHING AND COOLING DOWN

The Benefits of a Warm-Up

Warming up is essential. It reduces the risk of injury and eases your body into the workout that will come.

We'll be using a dynamic warm-up, which is a sequence of movements and stretches to help your joints get a greater range of motion. Warming up also allows more oxygen and blood flow to our muscles, which will then move better because they have the nutrients they need to perform, and your heart will be prepared for the workout.

Lastly, warming up is a signal to your mind and deepens your commitment to the process. It's a part of forming the routine that then forms the consistent habit, that then creates your results. So enjoy the warm-up and let it do all of the positive things to your whole body!

Cooldown Exercises

Like warming up, one common mistake people make with their workouts is not cooling down when they are done. A cooldown helps put your body into recovery mode and when you take the time to cool down, you delay the onset of muscle soreness, which tends to kick in one or two days after your workout.

Cooling down also helps to increase your flexibility. A cooldown is the optimal time to static stretch because your muscles are warm enough to endure holding it.

Pilates-Style Breathing

Breathing is something we do automatically, without a second thought, but breathing is really important in exercise. And I don't just mean being *able* to breathe, I mean breathing correctly!

Mindful Breathing

In Pilates, breathing correctly coordinates how the deep core muscles, pelvic floor, and diaphragm muscles work together. This is called mindful breathing and by doing it, you will achieve a full range of motion and get the best results from the exercises.

Also, mindful breathing helps us to focus and relax! It's done in a consistent rhythm, which can help to relax your mind, relieving anxiety and tension and in turn, increasing your mood and energy level. There's no better result, so look forward to the breathing exercises!

Get Support From a Chair, and Also Exercise While Sitting!

And finally, let's talk about using a chair as another way to implement support and add variety to your Pilates practice.

How many hours in a day do you think you are sitting? Between working, watching TV and

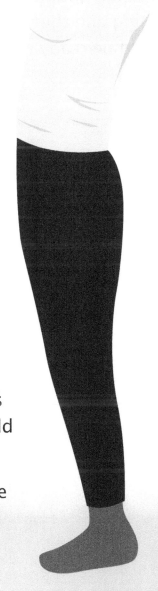

other leisurely activities, the amount of time we sit adds up quicker than we realize.

It's okay—because we can combat the sedentary hours by executing a few exercises *while* sitting.

Staying active, even if it's low impact and sitting, can help you achieve the fitness goals you have set for yourself. This means that you can practice Pilates from the comfort and support of a chair.

Throughout the 28-Day routine that follows, there are quite a number of exercises that incorporate a chair, so that you can get all the benefits of Pilates in multiple ways, and can also learn some exercises that you can do any time, even while watching TV!

Now, with all of this preparation for setting up your space, learning about mindful breathing and the importance of the warm up and cool down exercises, you should be ready to move into the routines!

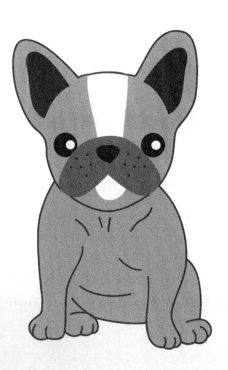

DOWNLOAD **FREE** BONUS MATERIALS!

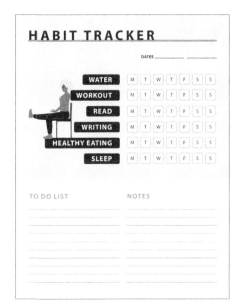

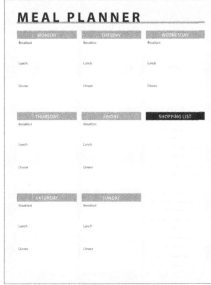

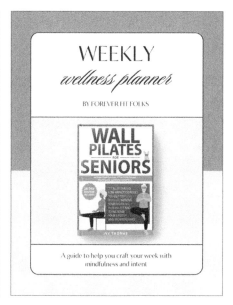

Habit Tracker

Meal Planner

Wellness Planner

Download these free materials to help set you up for success on your health journey. Watch as small changes lead to **BIG** results!

Scan the QR code and get your free companion materials to use throughout the book.

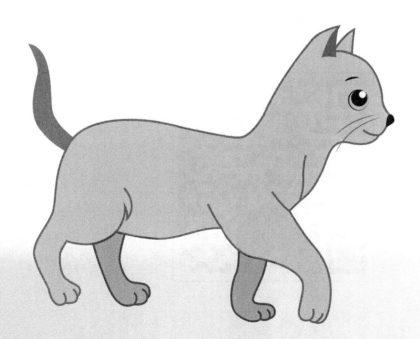

CHAPTER 4:

CUSTOMIZABLE 28-DAY ROUTINES FOR ALL LEVELS

You're ready! Here's a customizable 28-day plan that will take you approximately 15 minutes to start, and will work up to 30 or 40 minutes as you progress.

There's a mix of Wall Pilates and Chair Pilates, so have your sturdy chair handy, alongside your wall and yoga mat. This is where you'll also want to use your Habit Tracker!

Here's how the routines are structured for each day:
- Begin with mindful breathing
- 2 x warm-up exercises
- 2 x exercises
- Possible bonus / advanced exercise
- 2 x cooldown exercises
- Finish with mindful breathing again.

Start with the 28-Day routine as is, and build in the bonus / advanced exercises on your second 28-Day loop.

To build your exercise habit, the routine is designed to be done as a 28-Day loop on an on-going basis. Any bonus exercises are more challenging ones that are meant to be done during your second 28-day loop and beyond.

Listen to your body and work up to the suggested number of repetitions and sets of each exercise. There's also a rest day once a week.

This ultimately gives you a day-by-day workout that you can customize according to your fitness level, as you progress and solidify your exercise routine!

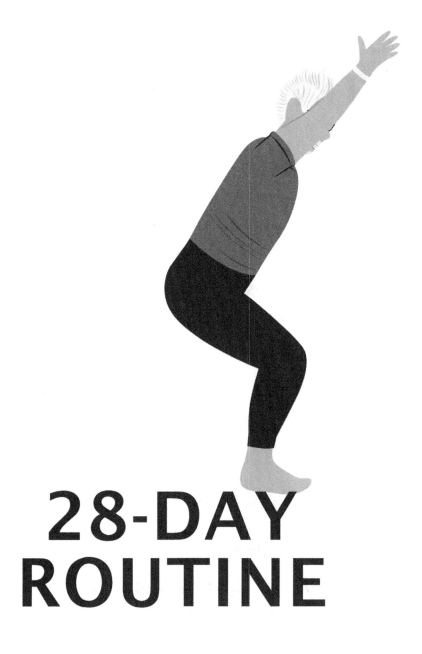

28-DAY
ROUTINE

WEEK ONE - DAY ONE

DEEP LATERAL BREATHING (IN A CHAIR)
1 minute

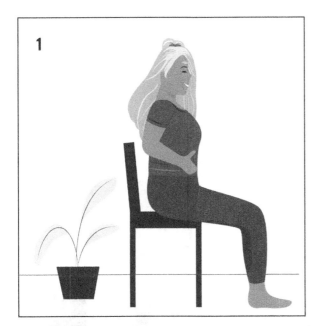 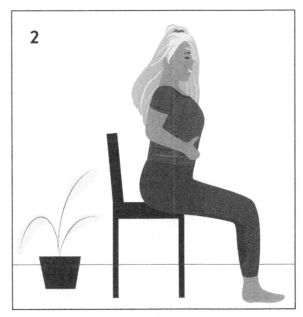

Breathing is so important, that this is an exercise that you'll start and end each daily routine with!

1. Sit comfortably on a chair with your hands on your waist near your rib cage.
2. Inhale deeply through your nose, allowing the air to move to your sides and back. Feel how your ribs expand with each breath as they push into your hands with each inhale.
3. Exhale through your mouth. You will feel your ribs contract or deflate, and your hands will move closer to one another.
4. Continue following this breathing pattern for a few minutes, feeling your ribs expand and contract more with each breath.

Lateral breathing contracts your abdominal muscles to stabilize your core. It also helps remove old air from your lungs and replaces it with fresh air, which helps to move more oxygen into your blood and improve your circulation.

Tip: Confine the breathing to your ribcage. Don't move your shoulders and ensure your neck and jaw are relaxed and neutral, and you that you maintain a straight spine.

NECK ROLLS

5 times in each direction

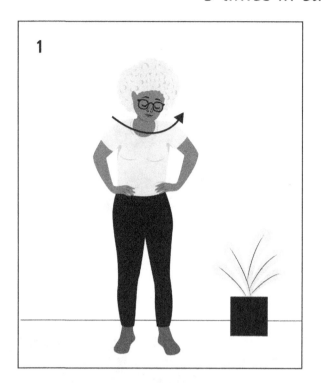 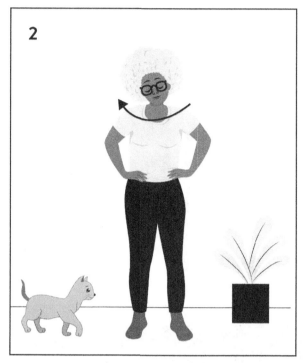

1. **Stand tall with your hands on your waist and your head facing forward. Ensure your shoulders are away from your ears and your core supports your posture.**

2. **Tuck your chin down towards your neck and slowly roll your head to the left, until your chin is above your left shoulder, and you're looking slightly upwards and behind you.**

3. **Drop your chin, and tuck it in as you slowly roll your head down and to the right, until your chin is above your right shoulder, and you're looking slightly upwards and behind you on the right side.**

4. **Repeat in alternating directions 5 times.**

Our necks are critical. This dynamic movement helps ease tense neck muscles while stretching them.

WEEK ONE - DAY ONE

ANKLE PUMPS
10 times with each ankle

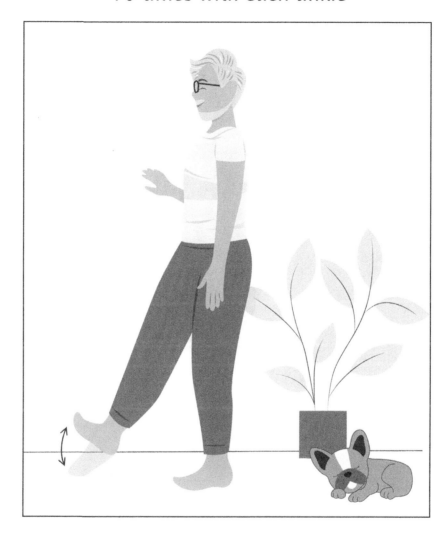

1. **Stand tall next to your wall with your right hand resting against it for support.**

2. **Extend your right leg with your heel a few inches above the floor.**

3. **Push your toes down (like you would on a gas pedal), hold for a few seconds, then bring your toes back up and toward your shin.**

4. **Repeat 10 times, then switch legs.**

Ankle pumps help to strengthen the ligaments and tendons in your joints. This exercise will also increase circulation to the area and your ankle's range of motion.

CALF RAISES
20 times

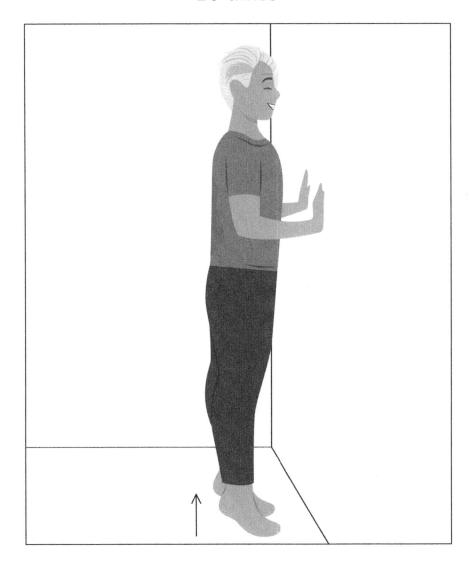

1. **Stand facing your wall with your feet about hip-width apart. Engage your core muscles to lengthen your spine. Your feet should be facing forward.**

2. **Lift your heels off the floor.**

3. **Lower and repeat up to 20 times.**

Strengthening your calves has plenty of benefits but, most importantly, having strong calves benefits your ankles and feet.

WALL SITS
Hold for 10 - 30 seconds

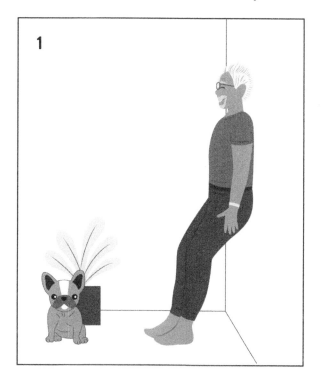
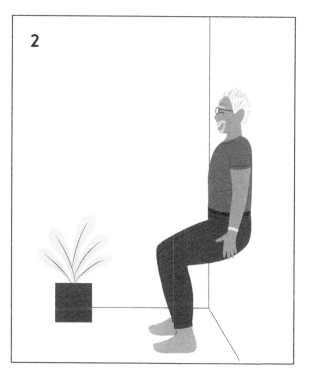

Wall sits are the holding position of a wall squat. You will stay squatted, as if you are sitting in an imaginary chair, and will hold that position for 10 - 30 seconds before you stand back up again.

1. **Stand with your back against the wall and your feet hip distance apart.**

2. **Step about two feet forward while keeping your back on the wall.**

3. **Engage your core muscles and slide down the wall as if you are about to sit on a stool or chair, ensuring your knees are stacked over your ankles and are not extending over your toes.**

4. **Hold for as long as possible (aim for at least 10 seconds, and work up to 30 seconds).**

This exercise, though challenging, will help build endurance and strength in your quads, glutes, calves, and core muscles. These muscles are critical to knee stability

WALL-ASSISTED QUAD STRETCH
Holding 30 seconds on each leg, 3 sets

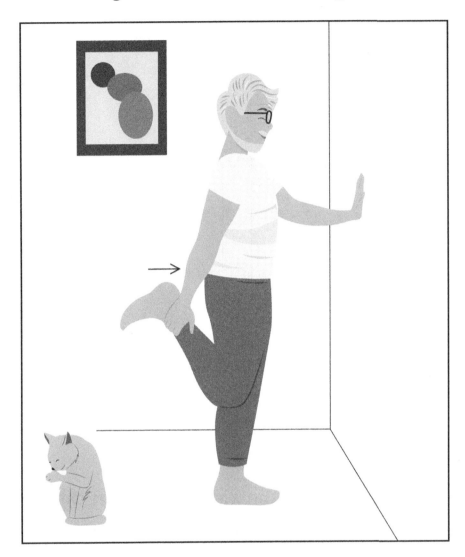

1. **Stand with your left hand against your wall.**

2. **Bend your right knee and grab your ankle with your right hand. Bring your heel as close to your bottom as possible until you feel a stretch in the front of your thigh.**

3. **Hold for 30 seconds.**

4. **Release, then switch legs. Do 3 sets.**

WALL-ASSISTED COBRA STRETCH
Holding for 20 seconds, 3 - 5 sets

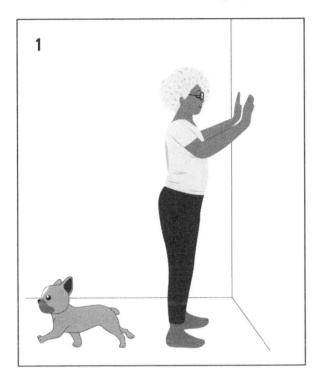 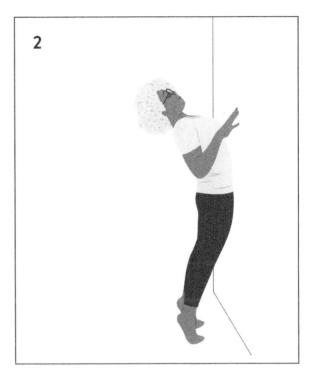

1. Stand an arm's length away from your wall, facing it.

2. Raise your hands to your shoulder height and rest them against the wall.

3. Press your hips forward to arch your back, lifting your chest to the ceiling. Tilt your gaze upwards.

4. Hold for 20 seconds, then relax and repeat three to five more times.

DEEP LATERAL BREATHING (IN A CHAIR)
1 minute

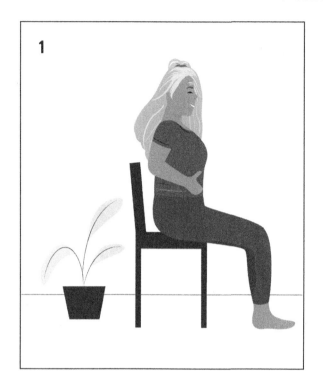 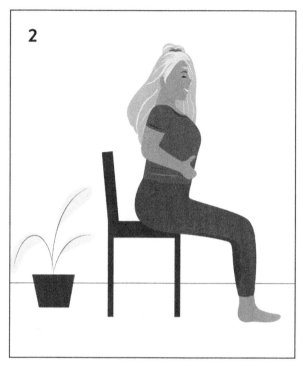

1. Sit comfortably on a chair with your hands on your waist near your rib cage.

2. Inhale deeply through your nose, allowing the air to move to your sides and back. Feel how your ribs expand with each breath as they push into your hands with each inhale.

3. Exhale through your mouth. You will feel your ribs contract or deflate, and your hands will move closer to one another.

4. Continue following this breathing pattern for a few minutes, feeling your ribs expand and contract more with each breath.

Lateral breathing contracts your abdominal muscles to stabilize your core. It also helps remove old air from your lungs and replaces it with fresh air, which helps to move more oxygen into your blood and improve your circulation.

NOTE: From here on out, you'll see a reminder banner to begin and end each day with your mindful breathing.

SHOULDER ROLLS
10 times in each direction

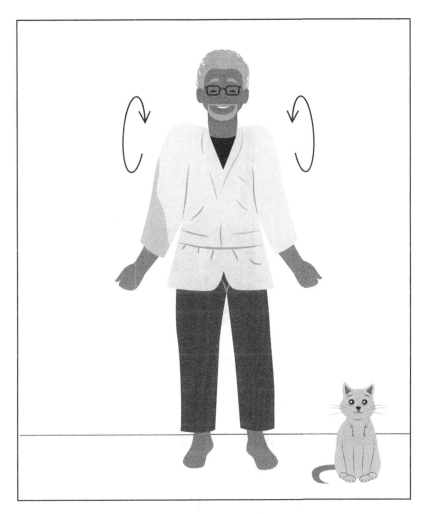

1. Stand with a tall spine and your feet about hip-width apart. Allow your hands to dangle by your sides.

2. Begin rolling your shoulders backward by lifting them toward your ears and then back. Continue until you have completed 10 rotations.

3. To roll your shoulders forward, you will begin by squeezing your shoulder blades and then lifting your shoulders toward your ears. Push your shoulders forward, then back down. Continue until you have completed 10 rotations.

SEATED ARM CIRCLES
10 times in each direction, 2 sets

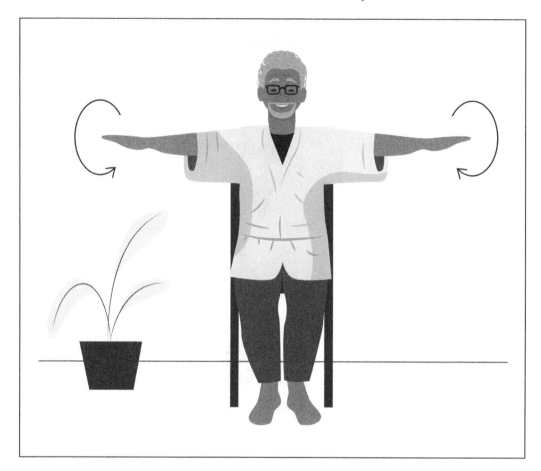

1. Sit in your chair with a lengthened spine. Ensure your core muscles are engaged.

2. Extend your arms to make a "T" shape with your palms facing the floor.

3. Start making small circles from your shoulder joint with your arms circling to the back. Continue doing this, making your circles larger each time for 30 seconds.

4. Lower your arms and shake them out.

5. Lift them back up to the "T" shape and repeat with your circles going to the front for 30 seconds.

6. Repeat 10 times in each direction and do 2 sets.

WALL ANGELS
8 to 10 times, 2 sets

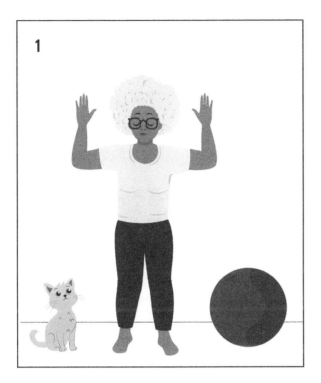 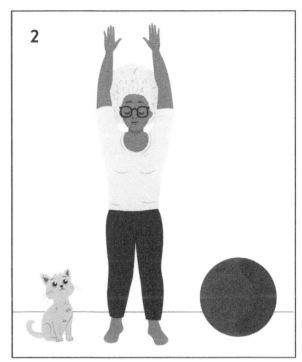

1. Stand about six inches from your wall with your back facing it.

2. Engage your core to straighten your spine.

3. Slightly bend your knees and lean against the wall, ensuring your head, torso, lower back and butt touch it.

4. Lift your arms to a 90 degree angle and open your shoulders. As you move your arms into this position, ensure your arms and elbows stay against the wall.

5. Slide your arms up the wall, keeping your arms and shoulders against the wall, until your hands are as high above your head as you can. Stretch your arms up even further by at least an inch and hold the position for 10 seconds.

6. Still keeping your arms and hands against the wall, slide your arms down until they're back in the starting position (with your elbows at 90 degrees and with your hands at the level of your shoulders). Repeat this 8 - 10 times and do 2 sets.

The point of doing wall angels is to open up your shoulders from the hunched forward position that a lot of us do during the day. The key is to keep your low back and shoulders up against the wall as you move your arms up, and then down. You should feel a stretch in your shoulders where you normally hunch forward.

WALL PUSH-UPS
5 - 10 times

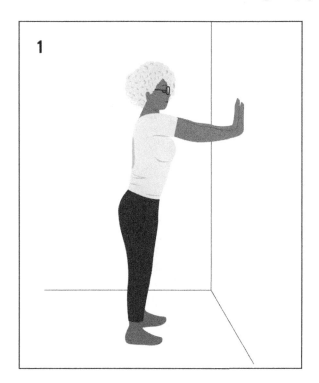 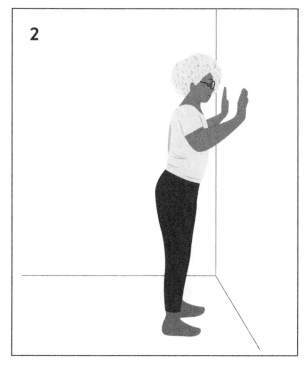

1. Stand no more than two feet from the wall, adjusting the distance according to your fitness level. You'll want to be closer to the wall if traditional push-ups are hard for you.

2. Place your hands on the wall at your shoulder height, just a bit wider than your shoulder width, and fingers are pointing up to the ceiling. Adjust your legs to be hip-width apart.

3. Engage your core and inhale.

4. Exhale to lower your chest toward the wall.

5. Inhale to push back up to the start and repeat.

6. Continue until you have completed 5 - 10 push-ups.

BONUS / ADVANCED EXERCISE

WEEK ONE - DAY TWO

CLOSE-GRIP WALL PUSHUPS
5-10 times

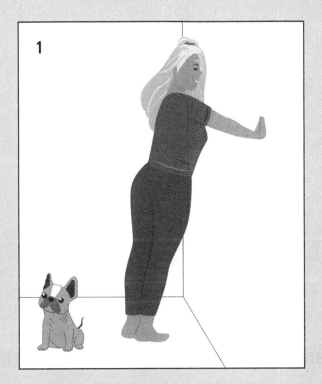 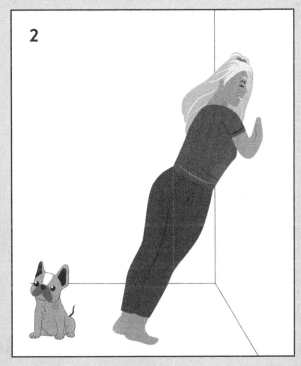

1. Begin by positioning your body as in the traditional wall pushup, with your hands slightly closer together (about 6 to 10 inches apart). Ensure your legs are hip-distance apart.

2. Inhale and engage your core.

3. Exhale as you lower your chest to the wall, keeping your elbows close to your body.

4. Inhale to push back up to the start and repeat.

WALL SHOULDER EXTENSION STRETCH
Hold for 20 seconds, 2 sets

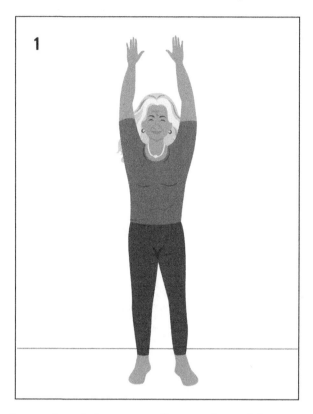 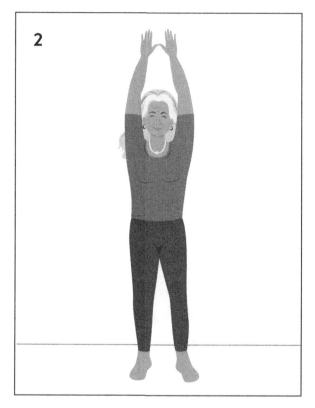

1. Stand with your feet shoulder-width apart and your back against the wall.

2. Extend your arms above your head with the backs of your hands resting against the wall.

3. Keeping your elbows straight, slide your hands up the wall until you feel a stretch in your shoulders.

4. Hold for 20 seconds. Do 2 sets.

SEATED ROLL-DOWN
5 times

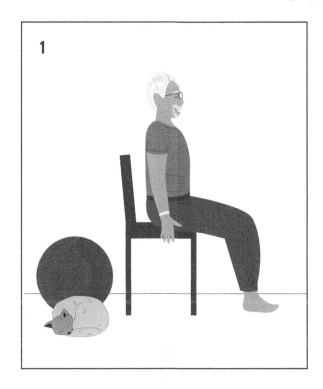

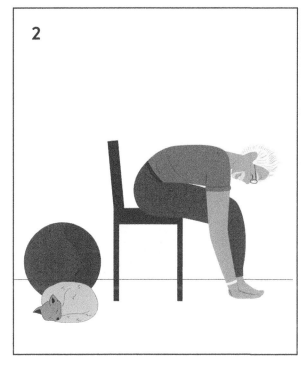

1. Sit near the edge of your seat and rest your hands at your side. Ensure your legs are about hip-width apart.

2. Inhale to engage your core muscles and lengthen your spine.

3. Exhale and slowly roll down, starting with tucking your chin into your chest to round your back and slowly roll down. Allow your hands to dangle in front of you or touch the floor when you are as far as you can go.

4. Hang out for as long as you need. When you are ready, inhale to slowly come back up, picturing your vertebrae stacking on one another as you go.

FINISH WITH 2 - 3 MINUTES OF DEEP LATERAL BREATHING Page 15

Page 15

3

BOXING PUNCHES
10 to 20 times on each side (or 1 minute)

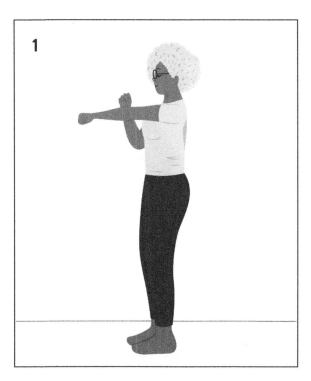

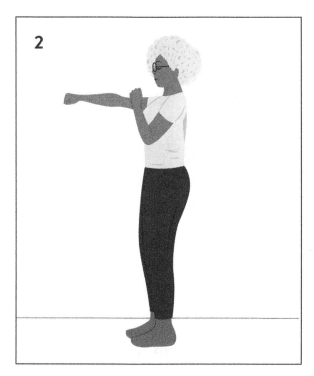

1. Stand with your feet about hip-width apart. Ensure your shoulders are down and away from your ears. Close your hands to make fists, bringing your arms in front of you like a boxer.

2. Punch your left arm out in front of you, then bring it back. Switch sides.

3. Repeat 10 to 20 times, or up to 1 minute.

Boxing punches are a cardio movement to help increase the circulation in your arms and even though you feel you're not moving too much, your heart rate will increase.

WRIST CIRCLES
30 seconds - 1 minute in each direction, 2 sets

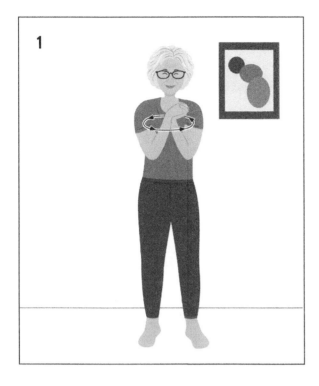 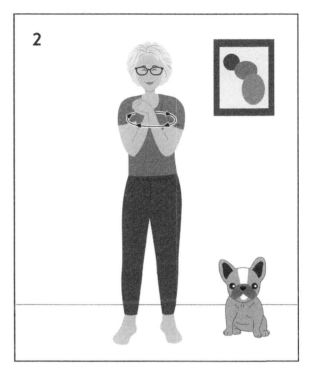

1. **Clasp your hands together, interlocking your fingers.**

2. **Rotate your wrists clockwise for 30 seconds to 1 minute. Then, switch directions. Do 2 sets.**

Our wrists are used more often than we realize every day. By performing wrist circles, you can help maintain your wrists' flexibility and range of motion.

TRADITIONAL WALL PLANK
Hold for 10 - 30 seconds

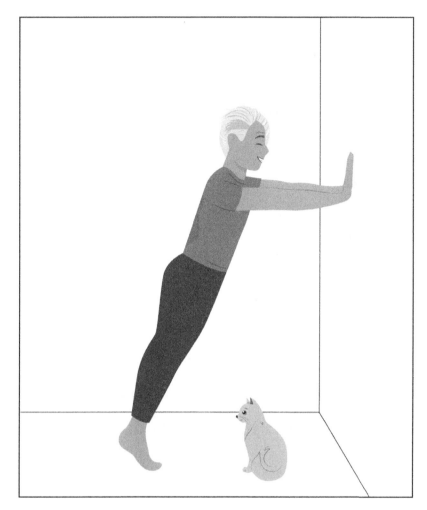

1. **Start with your hands resting against the wall, your arms straight, and your legs hip-width apart and slightly back from the wall to put your body in a straight diagonal.**
   To make this exercise more challenging, then instead of having your arms straight, bend them and rest your forearms against the wall.

2. **Engage your core and try to hold for as long as possible, but aim for at least 10 seconds and work up from there.**

Planks have plenty of benefits, especially for strengthening your core muscles. Using the wall will provide you with more stabilization for your core while helping you find a better balance.

WALL SQUAT WITH (OR WITHOUT) A STABILITY BALL
8 to 10 reps, 2 sets

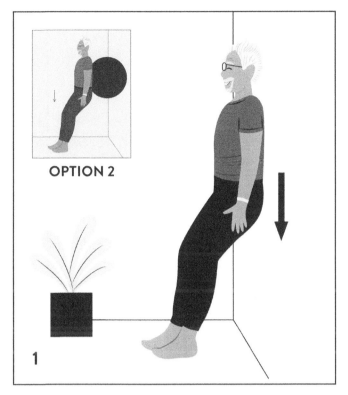
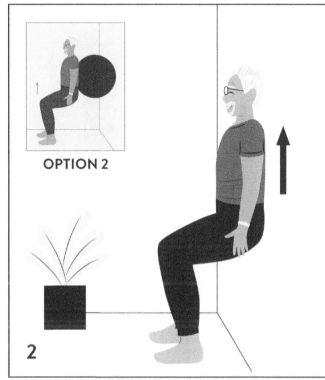

1. **If using the ball, place the ball between the curve of your lower back and the wall, resting your back on the ball. If you're not using the ball, simply rest your back on the wall itself.**

2. **Take a small step forward (about six inches).**

3. **Engage your core and inhale.**

4. **Exhale as you lower yourself, stopping when your knees are at a 90-degree angle.**

5. **Inhale as you stand back up.**

6. **Do 2 sets of 8 to 10 reps.**

If you are not feeling strong enough to execute a squat, a stability ball will be your new best friend. A stability ball can help you find proper form while supporting you through the movement. When choosing a stability ball, it's good to select one for your height. For example, if you're between 5' and 5'5", you'll want to select a ball that is 2 feet in diameter.

FORWARD BEND

1 time

3

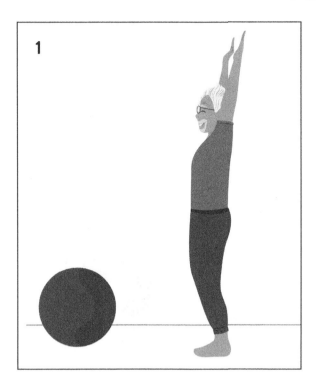
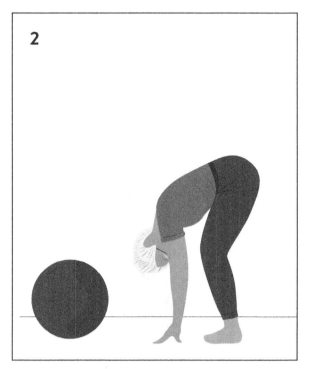

1. Stand with a straight spine and your feet about hip distance apart.

2. Reach your arms up overhead, then lower your arms down on both of your sides as you hinge at your hips to fold forward.

3. Aim to touch the floor if you can, but don't push yourself past what your body can comfortably do. Allow your head to hang as you breathe into the stretch.

4. Place your hands on your thighs or hips, and engage your core muscles to roll back up slowly one vertebrae at a time.

SEATED ROLL-DOWN
5 times

3

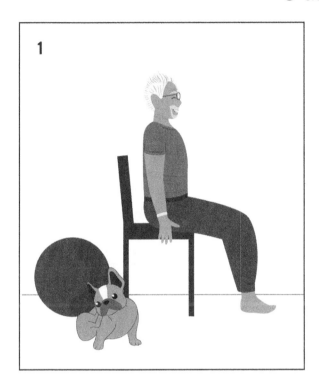

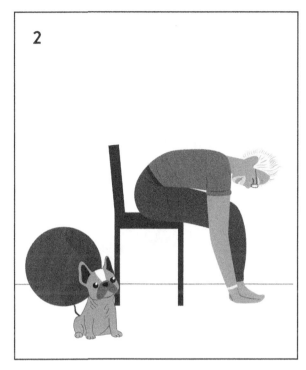

1. Sit near the edge of your seat and rest your hands at your side. Ensure your legs are about hip-width apart.

2. Inhale to engage your core muscles and lengthen your spine.

3. Exhale and slowly roll down, starting with tucking your chin into your chest to round your back and slowly roll down. Allow your hands to dangle in front of you or touch the floor when you are as far as you can go.

4. Hang out for as long as you need. When you are ready, inhale to slowly come back up, picturing your vertebrae stacking on one another as you go.

FINISH WITH 2 - 3 MINUTES OF DEEP LATERAL BREATHING Page **15**

4

LEG SWINGS
10 times with each leg

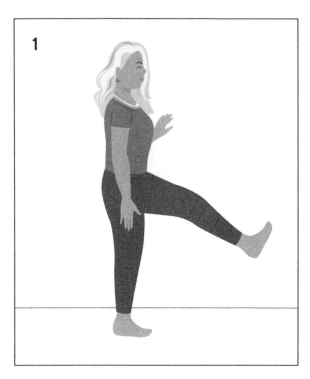

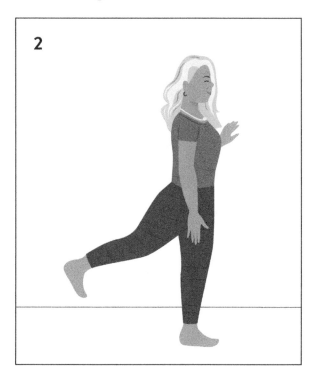

1. **Stand with your left side facing your wall. Engage your core muscles to keep you from losing your balance.**

2. **Keeping your left leg stationary, begin swinging your right leg forward and backward, aiming to swing higher each time.**

3. **Repeat 10 times in each direction, then switch sides.**

If you spend a significant amount of time sitting, it will impact your hip flexors because they become compressed. Over time, it can lead to pain and mobility issues. However, leg swings can help warm up and stretch the muscles and tendons in your hip joint, relieving any discomfort and removing your hips from a compressed position.

MARCHING
1 minute

4

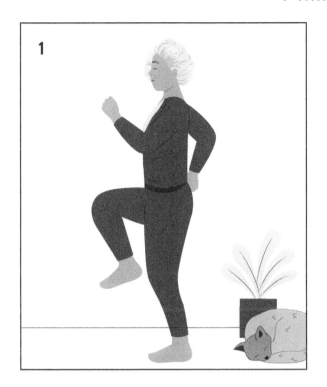 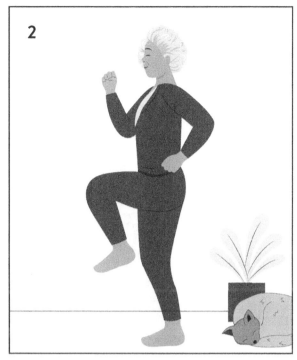

1. Stand with your feet hip-width apart. Engage your core muscles to straighten your spine. Your feet should be facing the front.

2. Lift your right leg as high as possible while simultaneously lifting your left arm with a bent elbow. Lower your leg and arm and repeat on the other side with your opposite arm and leg.

3. Continue alternating your legs until you've completed 12 to 15 on each side, or do up to 1 minute.

Get a boost of cardio with this warm-up exercise! Marching will help to boost your heart rate and increase the mobility and flexibility in your hips and quadriceps.

WALL SQUAT WITH (OR WITHOUT) A STABILITY BALL
8 to 10 reps, 2 sets

4

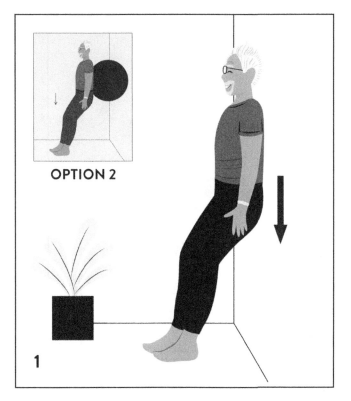

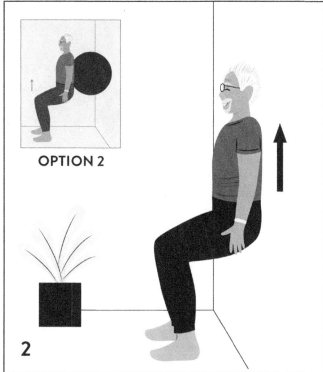

1. **If using the ball, place the ball between the curve of your lower back and the wall, resting your back on the ball. If you're not using the ball, simply rest your back on the wall itself.**

2. **Take a small step forward (about six inches).**

3. **Engage your core and inhale.**

4. **Exhale as you lower yourself, stopping when your knees are at a 90-degree angle.**

5. **Inhale as you stand back up.**

6. **Do 2 sets of 8 to 10 reps.**

If you are not feeling strong enough to execute a squat, a stability ball will be your new best friend. A stability ball can help you find proper form while supporting you through the movement. When choosing a stability ball, it's good to select one for your height. For example, if you're between 5' and 5'5", you'll want to select a ball that is 2 feet in diameter.

SEATED LEG CIRCLES

10 reps on each side, 2 sets

4

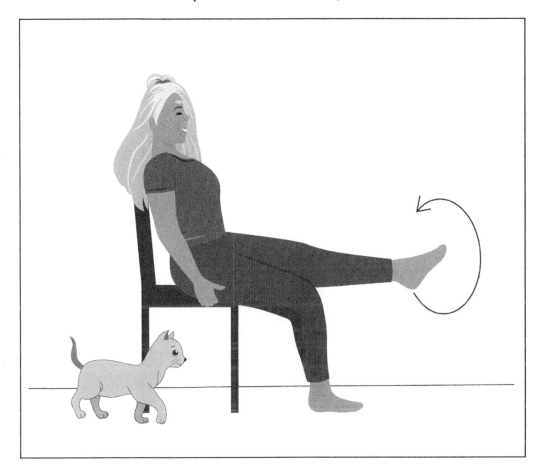

1. Sit forward in your chair, with your hands on the sides of the seat.

2. Lean into the back of the chair until your shoulders rest against your backrest. Keep your core engaged.

3. Extend your left leg to your hip's level.

4. Leading with your toes, slowly draw a large circle, then do it again going counterclockwise. Switch legs.

5. Continue alternating directions, both legs 10 times. Do 2 sets.

WALL-ASSISTED QUAD STRETCH
Holding 30 seconds on each leg, 3 sets

4

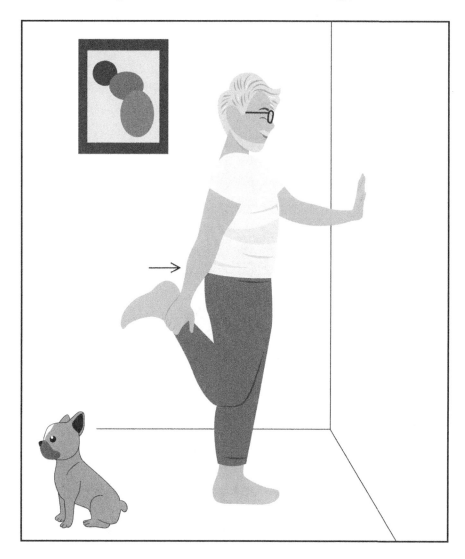

1. Stand with your left hand against your wall.

2. Bend your right knee and grab your ankle with your right hand. Bring your heel as close to your bottom as possible until you feel a stretch in the front of your thigh.

3. Hold for 30 seconds.

4. Release, then switch legs. Do 3 sets.

SEATED HIP FLEXOR STRETCH

Holding for 20 seconds, 2 sets

4

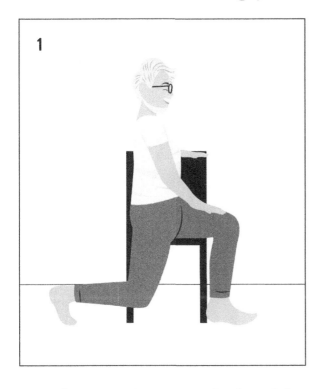

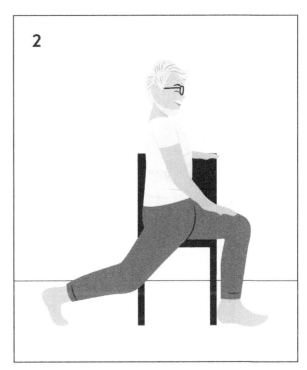

1. Sit sideways in your chair with your left side facing the backrest.

2. Extend your right leg as far behind you as possible until you feel a stretch in your hip and thigh. The ball of your foot should be placed flat on the floor, and your heel should be lifted. Ensure your spine is tall by engaging your core muscles.

3. Hold for 20 seconds.

4. Bring your leg back in, then switch sides. Do 2 sets.

FINISH WITH 2 - 3 MINUTES OF DEEP LATERAL BREATHING Page 15

BEGIN WITH 1 MINUTE OF DEEP LATERAL BREATHING Page 15

5

NECK ROLL AND STRETCH
5 times on each side

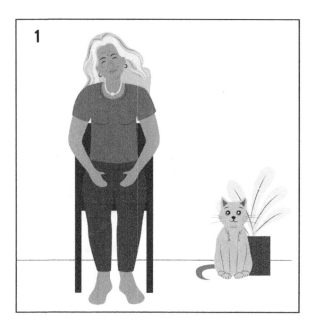

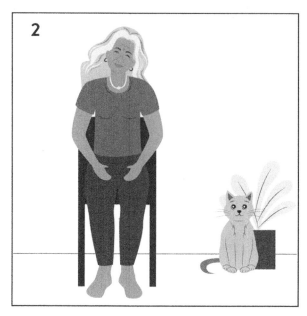

1. Sit in your chair with relaxed shoulders. Rest your hands on your lap.

2. Slowly tilt your head to the right to feel a stretch in the left side of your neck. Hold for a moment.

3. Gently roll your head forward while tucking in your chin to look down. Hold for a moment.

4. While keeping your chin tucked, turn your head to the right to look at your shoulder. Hold for a moment.

5. Turn your head back to the center to look back down at your lap, then bring your head back up to look forward.

6. Repeat on the left side.

7. Continue until you have completed this exercise five times on each side.

This exercise has a small rolling component, and will have you stretching the back of your neck as you roll it from right to left. It can be done standing or sitting in a chair. If you choose to stand, keep your legs about hip-width apart.

SHOULDER BLADE SQUEEZES
10 - 20 times

5

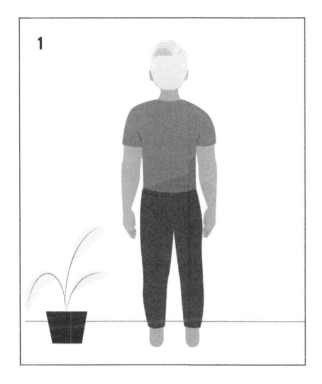 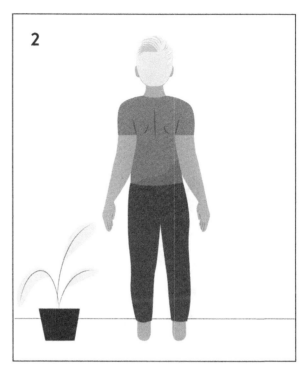

1. **Stand with a tall spine, feet about hip-width apart, and arms hanging by your sides.**

2. **Imagine a lemon between your shoulder blades as you pull your arms and elbows back to squeeze your shoulder blades together.**

3. **Release and repeat up to 20 times.**

Our shoulders are one of the most important joints in our upper body, however these joints are used too often, especially when lifting. Shoulder blade squeezes help maintain your joints' stability and improve your posture.

WALL SIDE LEG LIFTS
10 to 15 times on each side

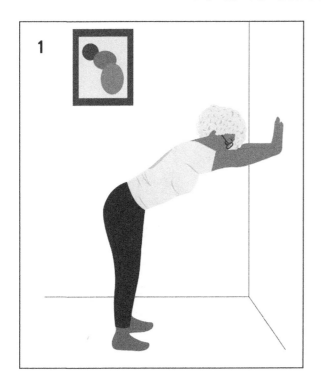
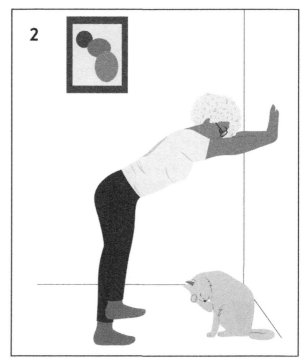

1. **Stand facing the wall.**

2. **Take a few steps back from the wall.**

3. **Bend forward to rest your hands on your wall for support. Your back should parallel the ceiling, and your toes should face the wall.**

4. **Engage your core and lift your leg to the side as high as it will go.**

5. **Lower it down halfway, then lift it back up.**

Leg lifts work your entire core muscles as you lift your legs to the side, including the ab muscles that make up our "six-pack" in the front, as well as our obliques, our back muscles, our diaphragm, our pelvic floor, our hip flexors and our glute (butt) muscles. In other words, these are great for us in all sorts of ways!

WALL SITS
Hold for 10 - 30 seconds

5

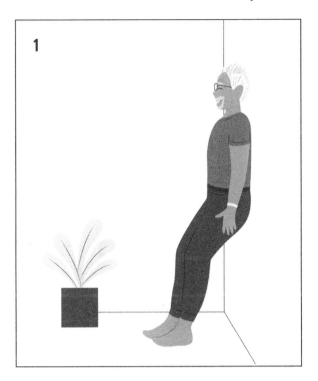 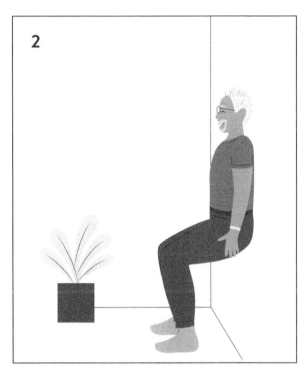

Wall sits are the holding position of a wall squat. You will stay squatted, as if you are sitting in an imaginary chair, and will hold that position for 10 - 30 seconds before you stand back up again.

1. **Stand with your back against the wall and your feet hip distance apart.**

2. **Step about two feet forward while keeping your back on the wall.**

3. **Engage your core muscles and slide down the wall as if you are about to sit on a stool or chair, ensuring your knees are stacked over your ankles and are not extending over your toes.**

4. **Hold for as long as possible (aim for at least 10 seconds, and work up to 30 seconds).**

This exercise, though challenging, will help build endurance and strength in your quads, glutes, calves, and core muscles. These muscles are critical to knee stability

SEATED HIP FLEXOR STRETCH

Holding for 20 seconds, 2 sets

5

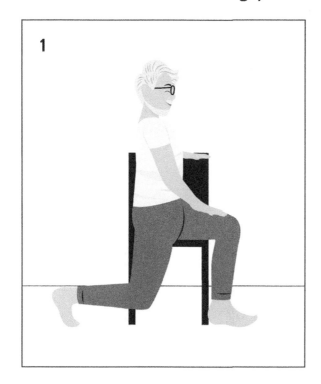

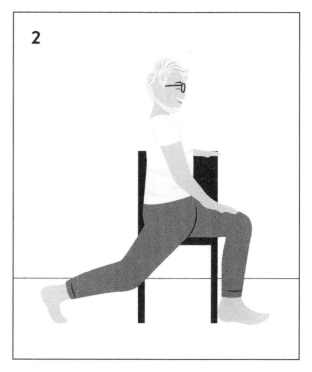

1. Sit sideways in your chair with your left side facing the backrest.

2. Extend your right leg as far behind you as possible until you feel a stretch in your hip and thigh. The ball of your foot should be placed flat on the floor, and your heel should be lifted. Ensure your spine is tall by engaging your core muscles.

3. Hold for 20 seconds.

4. Bring your leg back in, then switch sides. Do 2 sets.

SEATED ROLL-DOWN
5 times

5

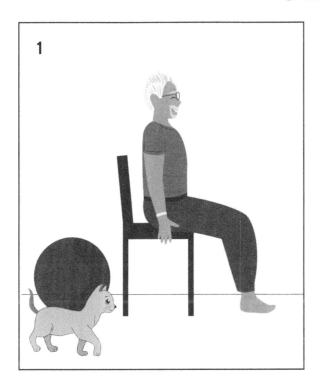 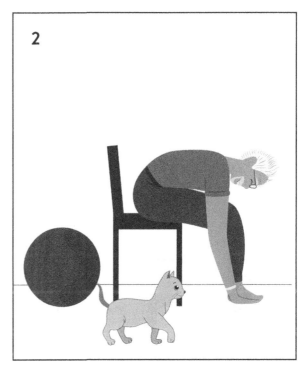

1. Sit near the edge of your seat and rest your hands at your side. Ensure your legs are about hip-width apart.

2. Inhale to engage your core muscles and lengthen your spine.

3. Exhale and slowly roll down, starting with tucking your chin into your chest to round your back and slowly roll down. Allow your hands to dangle in front of you or touch the floor when you are as far as you can go.

4. Hang out for as long as you need. When you are ready, inhale to slowly come back up, picturing your vertebrae stacking on one another as you go.

FINISH WITH 2 - 3 MINUTES OF DEEP LATERAL BREATHING Page 15

BEGIN WITH 1 MINUTE OF DEEP LATERAL BREATHING Page 15

SEATED MARCHES
1 minute

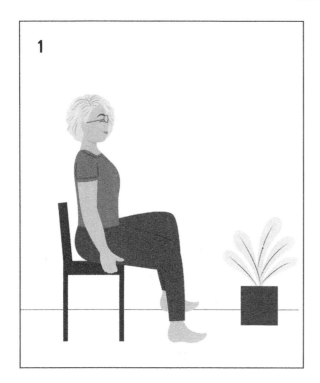

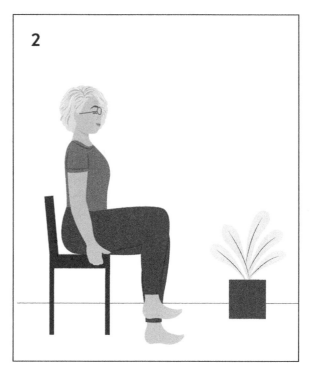

1. Sit in your chair near the front with your hands holding the sides of the seat for support.

2. Engage your core muscles to lengthen your spine.

3. Start lifting your left leg off the floor, then switch to your right in a marching movement.

4. Continue to march for a minute.

Seated marches will give you a quick boost of energy and cardio as they increase your heart rate. This exercise is great for a warm-up or any time during the day for movement.

HIGH KNEES
10 to 20 times on each side

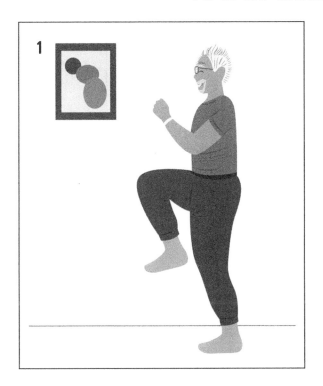 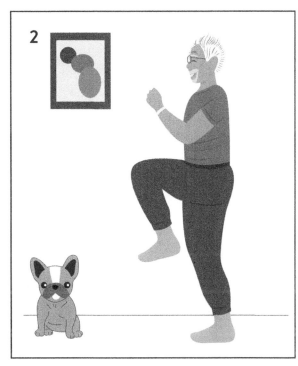

1. Stand with your feet shoulder-width apart and a tall spine. Ensure your shoulders are back and down, away from your ears. Have your elbows bent 90 degrees.

2. Bring your right knee up as high as possible, then switch legs.

3. Repeat until you have done 10 to 20 on each side.

CALF RAISES
20 times

6

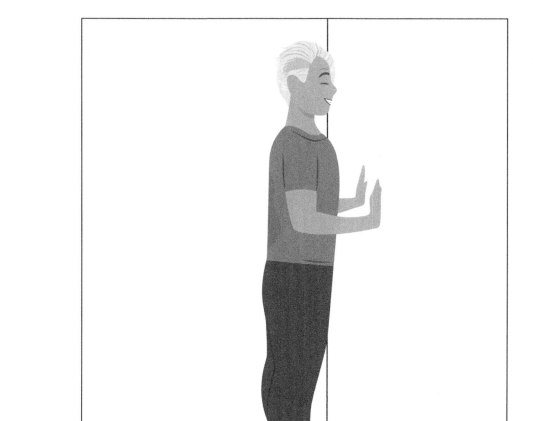

1. **Stand facing your wall with your feet about hip-width apart. Engage your core muscles to lengthen your spine. Your feet should be facing forward.**

2. **Lift your heels off the floor.**

3. **Lower and repeat up to 20 times.**

Strengthening your calves has plenty of benefits but, most importantly, having strong calves benefits your ankles and feet.

REVERSE LUNGES
10 reps on each side, 2 sets

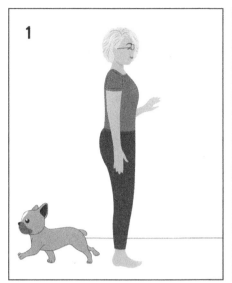 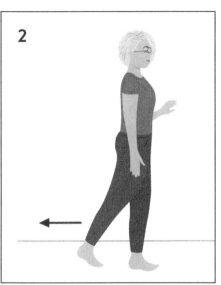 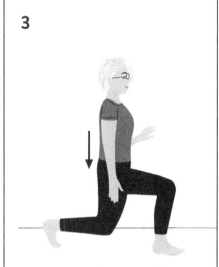

1. **Stand with your left side facing the wall. Rest your left hand against the wall and position your legs about hip-width apart.**

2. **Step back with your right leg and bend both knees until about 90 degrees. Your right knee should hover above the ground with your shin parallel to the floor.**

3. **Press into your left heel to straighten your leg, return your right leg to the starting position, and repeat.**

Lunges are great for strengthening our knees because they work your glutes and quads. That said, reverse lunges are sometimes preferable for knee injuries due to the decreased stress on your knee. It's also sometimes easier to maintain stability going backward instead of forwards.

WALL-ASSISTED HAMSTRING STRETCH
Holding 20 seconds, at least 3 times

6

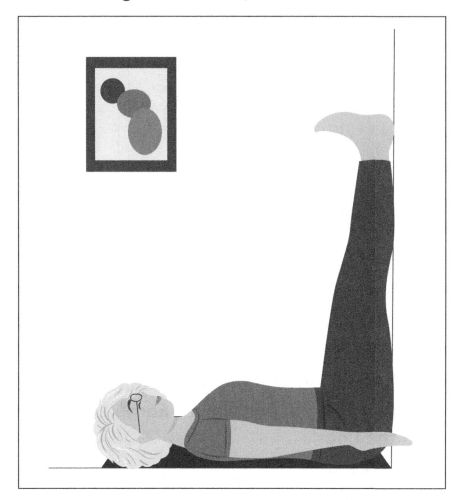

1. Lie in front of your wall with your legs resting against it, extended upwards toward the ceiling.

2. Shimmy your bottom close to the wall.

3. Press your heels into the wall as you straighten your knee until you feel a stretch in your hamstrings.

4. Hold for 20 seconds, then relax. Repeat at least 3 times or more if you can.

NOTE: This is one of the few exercises from the floor. If you don't feel up to it, then an alternate would be the Seated Heel Slides on p.107.

SEATED HIP FLEXOR STRETCH

Holding for 20 seconds, 2 sets

6

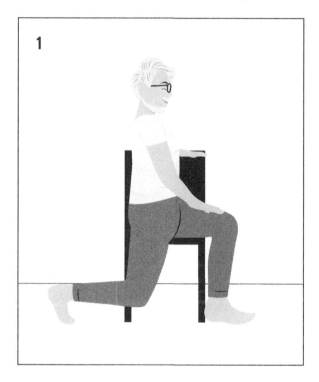 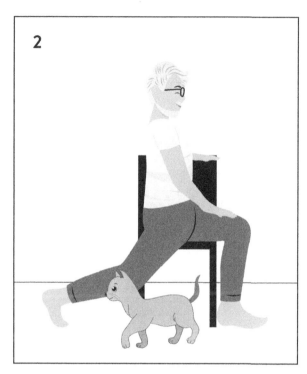

1. Sit sideways in your chair with your left side facing the backrest.

2. Extend your right leg as far behind you as possible until you feel a stretch in your hip and thigh. The ball of your foot should be placed flat on the floor, and your heel should be lifted. Ensure your spine is tall by engaging your core muscles.

3. Hold for 20 seconds.

4. Bring your leg back in, then switch sides. Do 2 sets.

FINISH WITH 2 - 3 MINUTES OF DEEP LATERAL BREATHING Page 15

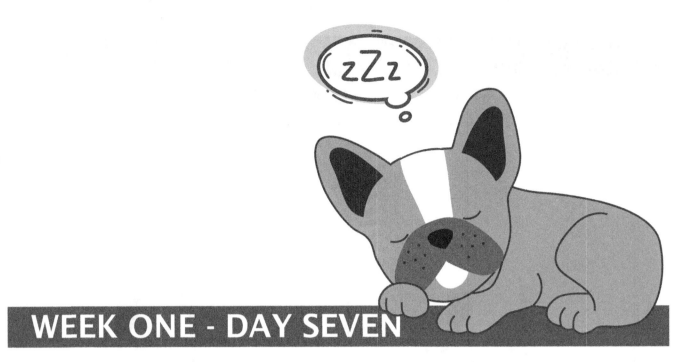

7

WEEK ONE - DAY SEVEN

REST DAY

ENJOYING THIS BOOK?

If so, please consider leaving a review  !

I value your feedback and would greatly appreciate it if you could take a moment to share your thoughts with me publicly. Your thoughts ensure that I continue to meet and exceed yours and others' expectations, who are seeking high quality information and a great experience!

US CUSTOMERS, SCAN QR CODE:

GLOBAL CUSTOMERS, FOLLOW THESE STEPS:

1. Go to your Amazon "Your Orders" page ("Digital Orders" if you purchased the e-book)

2. Select "Wall Pilates for Seniors" by Ivy Thomas

3. Click on "WRITE A PRODUCT REVIEW" and describe your experience of this book.

AND THANK YOU!

BEGIN WITH 1 MINUTE OF DEEP LATERAL BREATHING Page 15

LEG SWINGS
10 times with each leg

8

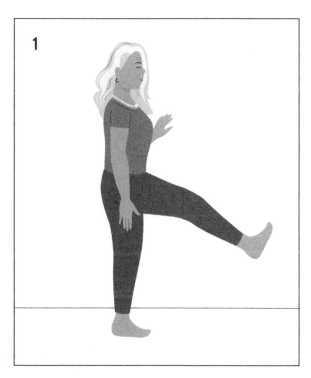

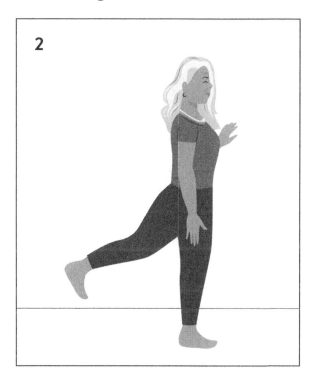

1. **Stand with your left side facing your wall. Engage your core muscles to keep you from losing your balance.**

2. **Keeping your left leg stationary, begin swinging your right leg forward and backward, aiming to swing higher each time.**

3. **Repeat 10 times in each direction, then switch sides.**

If you spend a significant amount of time sitting, it will impact your hip flexors because they become compressed. Over time, it can lead to pain and mobility issues. However, leg swings can help warm up and stretch the muscles and tendons in your hip joint, relieving any discomfort and removing your hips from a compressed position.

HIGH KNEES
10 to 20 times on each side

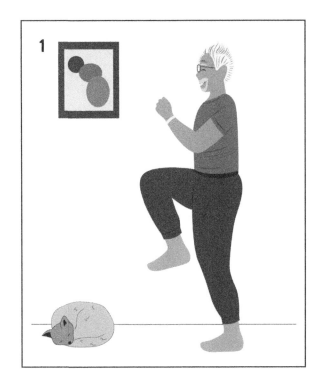 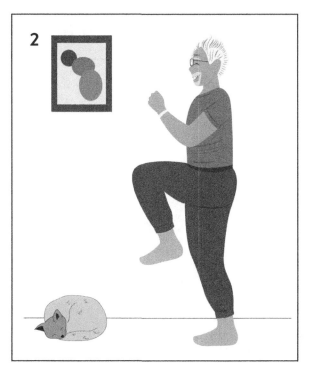

1. Stand with your feet shoulder-width apart and a tall spine. Ensure your shoulders are back and down, away from your ears. Have your elbows bent 90 degrees.

2. Bring your right knee up as high as possible, then switch legs.

3. Repeat until you have done 10 to 20 on each side.

WALL LUNGES

8 to 10 times on each side

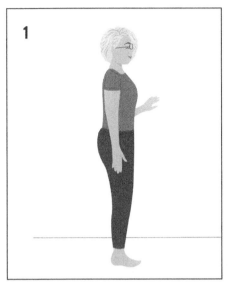 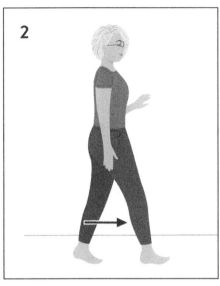 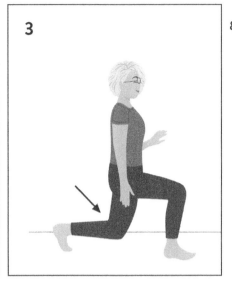

1. Stand with your left side facing the wall and rest your hand on it for support. Ensure your shoulders are back and away from your ears, and you lean forward slightly.

2. Engage your core and step back with your left leg while bending your left knee to about 90 degrees.

3. Press into your right leg to come back to standing.

4. Continue until you have completed between 8 and 10 reps, then switch legs.

Lunges, in general, are great for strengthening our knees because they work your glutes and quads.

NOTE: If this is too hard or causes any knee pain, consider doing a Reverse Lunge on p.51.

SINGLE-LEG WALL SQUAT
WITH (OR WITHOUT) STABILITY BALL
10 times, 2 sets

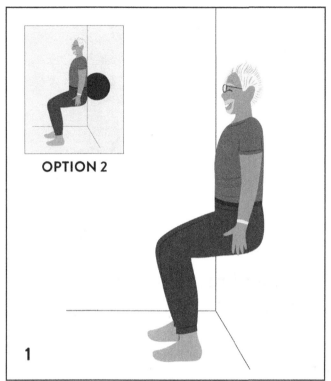

OPTION 2

1

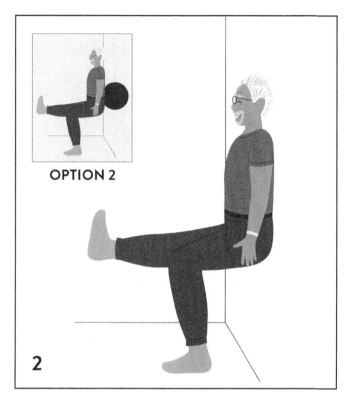

OPTION 2

2

1. Stand with your back against the wall.

2. Shift your weight to your left leg and then lift your right leg so that it's in front of you, with your foot flexed and pointing up to the ceiling.

3. Engage your core to lengthen your spine.

4. Press your back into the stability ball as you inhale.

5. Exhale and lower into the squat with your right leg.

6. Inhale to stand back up and repeat 10 times. Do 2 sets.

NOTE: If this is too hard, just lift your right foot so that it's simply off the floor.

BONUS EXERCISE

WEEK TWO - DAY ONE

CHAIR SQUATS
5 reps

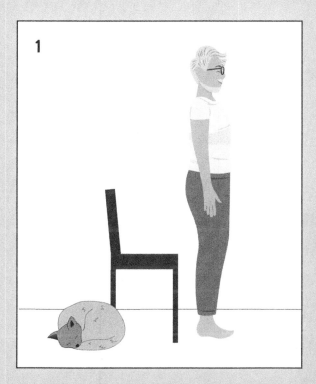
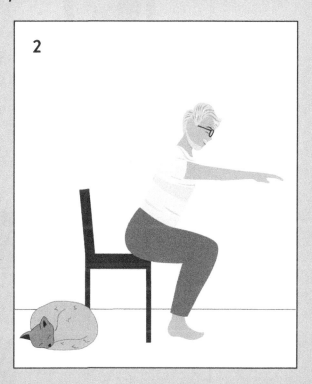

1. **Stand slightly in front of your chair, facing away. Have your legs about shoulder-width apart with your toes facing the front.**

2. **Engage your core and move your shoulders away from your ears.**

3. **Begin to bend your knees and lower your bottom down to the seat. Lift your arms in front of you for balance if you need to.**

4. **Stop when your bottom touches the seat, then stand back up.**

5. **Repeat for 5 times and work up to 2 sets.**

If you find wall squats challenging, a chair will become your best friend for perfecting the exercise. **Ensure your chair has no wheels.**

WALL-ASSISTED QUAD STRETCH

Holding 30 seconds on each leg, 3 sets

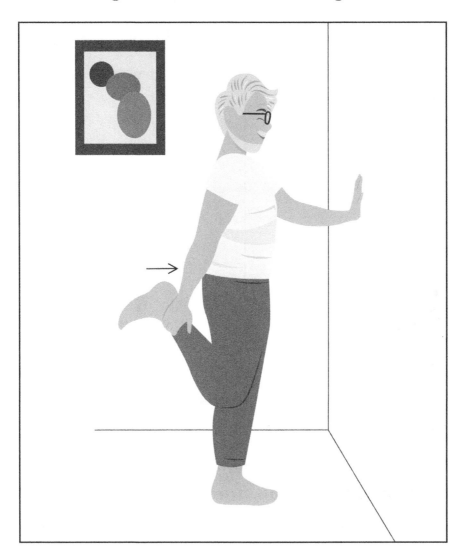

1. Stand with your left hand against your wall.

2. Bend your right knee and grab your ankle with your right hand. Bring your heel as close to your bottom as possible until you feel a stretch in the front of your thigh.

3. Hold for 30 seconds.

4. Release, then switch legs. Do 3 sets.

WALL ROLL-DOWNS
5 times

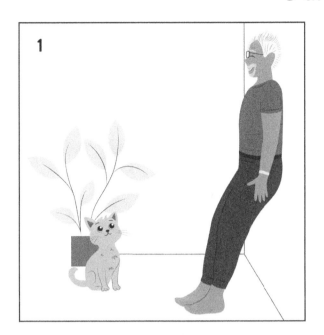 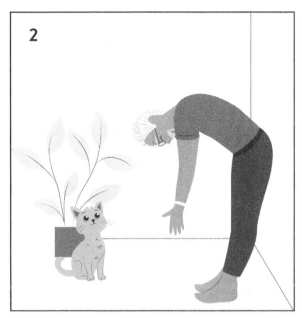

1. Stand with your back against the wall, ensuring your butt touches it. Have your feet about 6 to 10 inches from the wall. Your arms should dangle beside you with your shoulders away from your ears.

2. Engage your core muscles as you inhale deeply.

3. Exhale and slowly nod your head as you slowly roll down as far as possible. Ensure your butt stays on the wall while your upper back moves away. Your arms should also hang as you roll down; allow them, along with your head, neck, and shoulders, to relax. You may also want to scoop your abs in further to engage them as you roll down.

4. When you reach your furthest point, take another inhale. Feel how your back is curved between your torso's upper, middle, and lower sections. You may also feel a stretch in your hamstrings.

5. Exhale and slowly roll back up, picturing your vertebrae stacking on top of one another. Engage your abs to assist you as you go. Repeat 5 times.

FINISH WITH 2 - 3 MINUTES OF DEEP LATERAL BREATHING Page 15

BEGIN WITH 1 MINUTE OF DEEP LATERAL BREATHING

SEATED MERMAID
10 times on each side

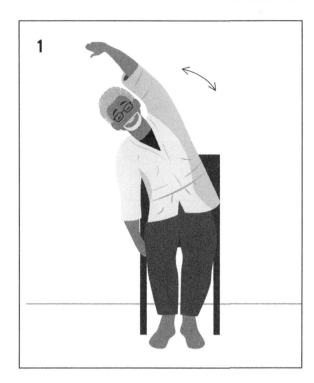

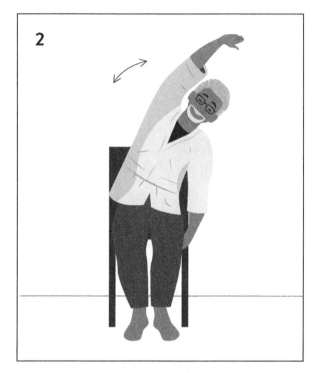

1. Sit in your chair with your legs about hip-width apart. Ensure your shoulders are back and down.

2. Place your right hand on the side of your chair as you reach your left arm overhead. Stretch to the right side until your left side feels a gentle stretch.

3. Hold the stretch and breathe into your ribcage. Return to the starting position on your last inhale and repeat on the right side.

4. Continue until you have completed 10 reps on each side.

ANKLE CIRCLES
5 times on each side

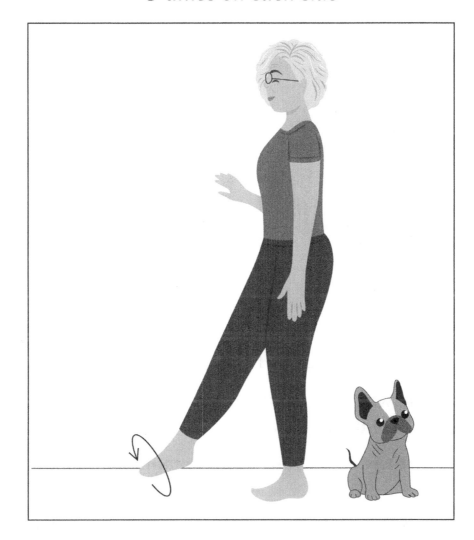

1. **Stand tall next to your wall with your right hand resting against it for support.**

2. **Extend your right leg with your heel a few inches above the floor.**

3. **Make circles with your foot clockwise 10 times, then counterclockwise.**

4. **Switch legs.**

5. **Repeat 5 times in each direction.**

Like our wrists, ankles are an essential joint in our body, as they help to support our body weight. Ankle circles will help to keep your ankles flexible, stable, and mobile.

WALL SQUATS WITH HEEL RAISES

8 to 10 times, 2 sets

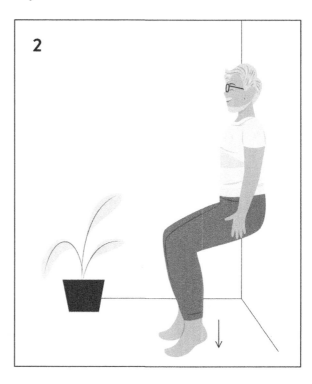

1. **Lean against the wall with your knees bent. Walk them out until you are "sitting" on an invisible chair.**

2. **Engage your core to ensure your back remains straight and flat against the wall.**

3. **Shift your weight to the balls of your feet to lift your heels.**

4. **Hold for three seconds, then lower, and stand back up.**

5. **Repeat steps three and four, 8 - 10 times. Do 2 sets.**

The wall squat combined with a heel raise targets all of the muscles a traditional squat does but with a twist. In this squat variation, raising your heels will further activate your quads as your knees will extend more over your toes in the squat position, aiding you to go just a little deeper.

TRADITIONAL WALL PLANK
Hold for 10 - 30 seconds

9

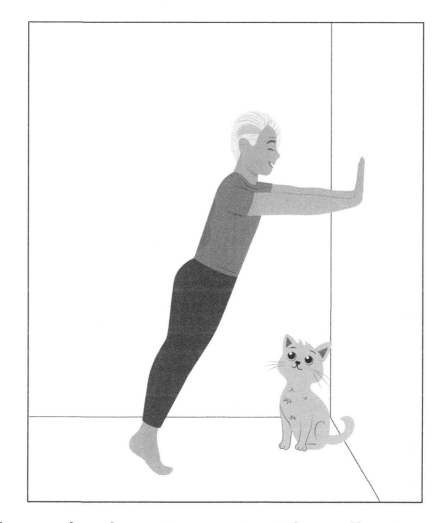

1. **Start with your hands resting against the wall, your arms straight, and your legs hip-width apart and slightly back from the wall to put your body in a straight diagonal.**
To make this exercise more challenging, then instead of having your arms straight, bend them and rest your forearms against the wall.

2. **Engage your core and try to hold for as long as possible, but aim for at least 10 seconds and work up from there.**

Planks have plenty of benefits, especially for strengthening your core muscles. Using the wall will provide you with more stabilization for your core while helping you find a better balance.

BONUS EXERCISE

WALL PLANK WITH LEG LIFT
10 to 20 reps

9

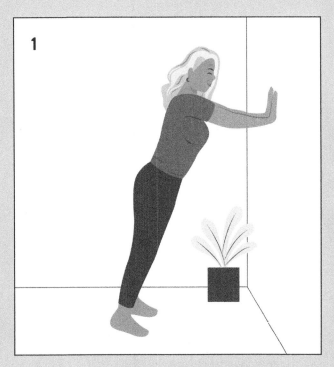 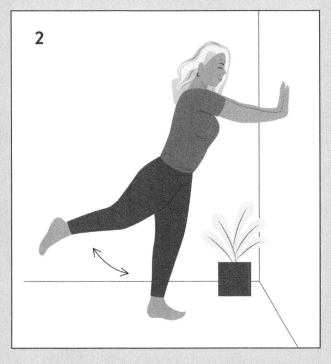

1. Start with your hands resting against the wall, your arms straight, and your legs hip-width apart and slightly back from the wall to put your body in a straight diagonal.

2. Ensuring your core is engaged, lift your right leg off the floor. Keep your foot flexed and your leg straight.

3. Continue to raise your leg until it's parallel to the floor (or as high as comfortable).

4. Hold your leg up for a few seconds, then slowly lower it back down.

5. Repeat with your left leg.

6. Continue alternating your legs until you've completed 10 to 20 leg lifts on each side.

WALL-ASSISTED CALF STRETCH
Hold for 20 seconds on each side

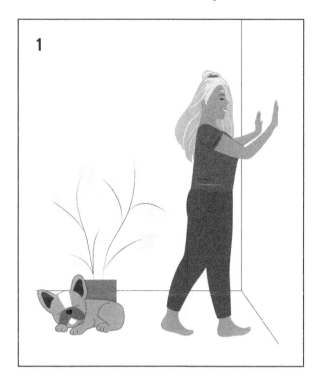 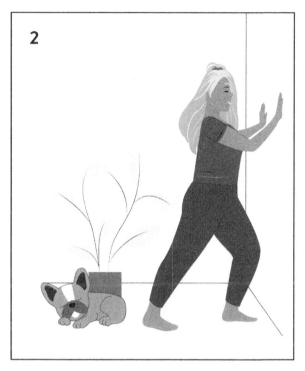

1. Stand an arm's length away from the wall, facing it.

2. Rest your hands against the wall at shoulder height.

3. Step your right foot back and bend your left leg. Ensure your right heel stays on the ground. If you can't get your heel onto the floor, shorten the distance.

4. Hold the stretch for 20 seconds, then switch legs.

WALL-ASSISTED SIDE BEND

Hold for 20 seconds on each side

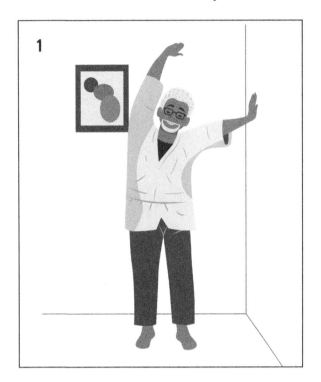
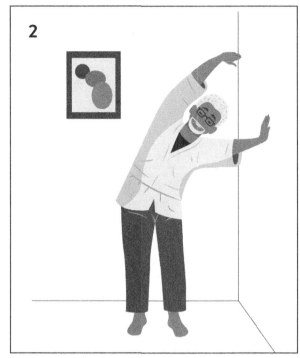

1. Stand with your left side facing the wall and your legs hip-distance apart.

2. Raise your left arm to shoulder height and rest your left hand against the wall.

3. Raise your right arm over your head, and stretch it as far as you can towards the wall.

4. Hold for 20 seconds. You should feel the stretch along the length of your right side, as well as a crunch in your left side abdomen muscles.

5. Switch sides and do the same stretch, holding for 20 seconds.

FINISH WITH 2 - 3 MINUTES OF DEEP LATERAL BREATHING Page 15

BOXING PUNCHES
10 to 20 times on each side (or 1 minute)

10

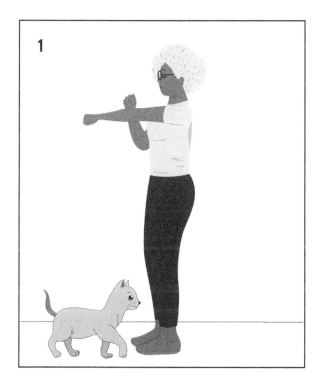

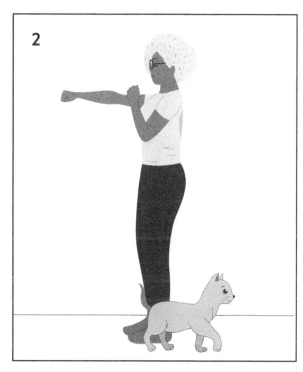

1. Stand with your feet about hip-width apart. Ensure your shoulders are down and away from your ears. Close your hands to make fists, bringing your arms in front of you like a boxer.

2. Punch your left arm out in front of you, then bring it back. Switch sides.

3. Repeat 10 to 20 times, or up to 1 minute.

Boxing punches are a cardio movement to help increase the circulation in your arms and even though you feel you're not moving too much, your heart rate will increase.

TORSO TWISTS
1 minute

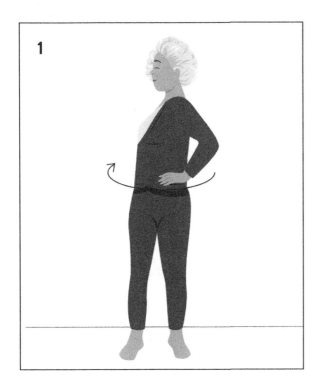

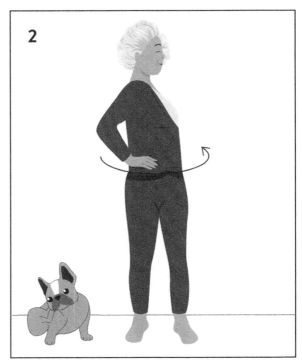

1. Stand tall with your feet hip-width apart and your hands on your waist.

2. Keeping your feet planted, twist your torso to the right as far as you can go, then twist the other way. Engage your core muscles and keep your feet planted on the floor so that the stretch is focused on your torso.

3. Repeat 5 to 10 times in each direction, or do more for up to a full minute.

WALL PELVIC TILT
10 times, 2 sets

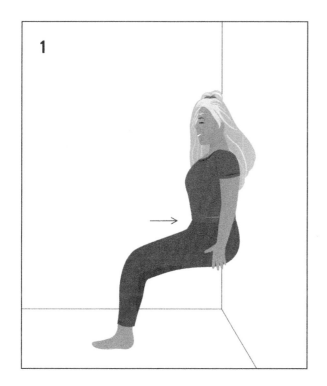 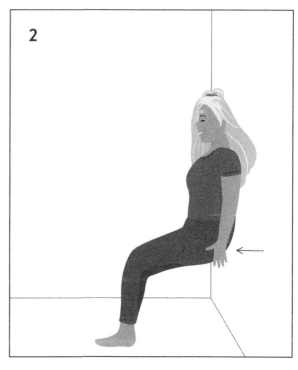

10

1. Stand facing away from the wall and lean your back to rest against it. Ensure your knees have a slight bend to them.

2. Take a deep inhale.

3. On the exhale, tilt your pelvis up and away from the wall, straightening the natural curve of your lower back. You may find your lower back touches the wall, which is good. That's the goal of the tilt.

4. Tilt your pelvis to return to the starting position on your next inhale.

5. Repeat 10 times and do 2 sets.

A pelvic tilt exercise can help address issues with your posture which can decrease back pain and strengthen your core.

TRADITIONAL WALL PLANK
Hold for 10 - 30 seconds

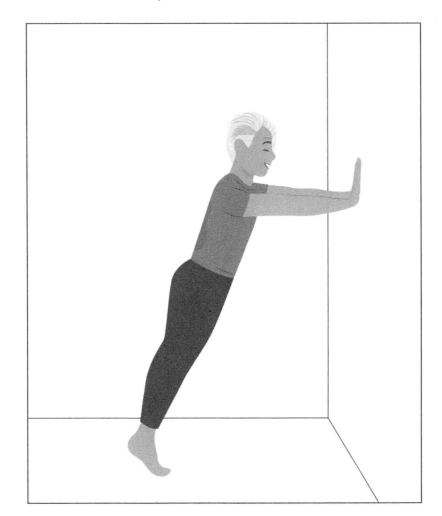

10

1. **Start with your hands resting against the wall, your arms straight, and your legs hip-width apart and slightly back from the wall to put your body in a straight diagonal.**
   To make this exercise more challenging, then instead of having your arms straight, bend them and rest your forearms against the wall.

2. **Engage your core and try to hold for as long as possible, but aim for at least 10 seconds and work up from there.**

Planks have plenty of benefits, especially for strengthening your core muscles. Using the wall will provide you with more stabilization for your core while helping you find a better balance.

BONUS EXERCISE

WEEK TWO - DAY THREE

WALL PLANK WITH SHOULDER TAP
10 to 20 reps on each side

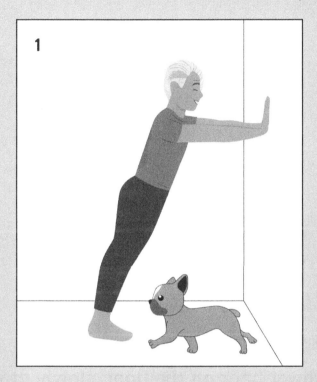 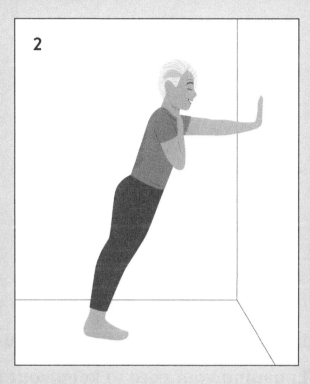

1. Start in the traditional wall plank position.

2. Engage your core to keep your body straight and unmovable.

3. Lift your right hand to tap your left shoulder. Return it to the wall and switch hands.

4. Continue to alternate hands until you've completed 10 to 20 shoulder taps on each side.

FLOOR WINDMILL BACK TWIST

3 times on each side

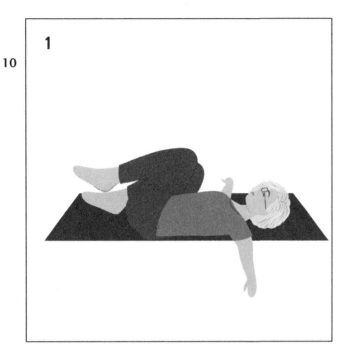
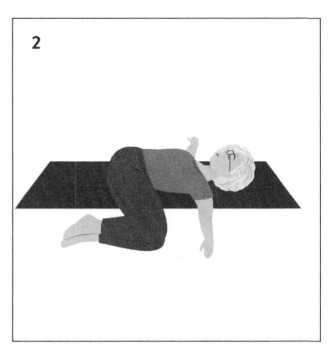

10

1. Lie down on your yoga mat with your knees bent.

2. Lift your feet off the floor so your shins are parallel to the ceiling.

3. Engaging your core to keep your lower back on the floor, slowly drop your knees to the right and hold for up to 20 seconds.

4. Engage your core to bring your legs back up and drop them to the other side.

5. Repeat each side 3 times.

This is one of the few exercises in this book where you'll need to be on the floor. However, working through the twisting motions will benefit your spine and release any tension.

Tip: Place your hands underneath your bottom if your lower back is coming off the floor.

NOTE: If you don't feel up to getting down on the floor, move to the next cooldown exercise and try to do more reps.

SEATED SPINAL TWISTS

2 times on each side

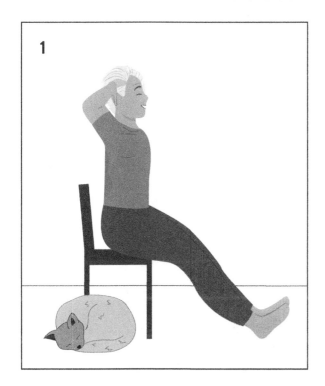

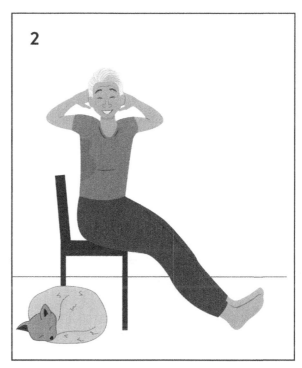

10

1. Sit in the center of your chair. Engage your core to lengthen your spine. Have your legs slightly wider than your hips.

2. Place your hands on the back of your head with your elbows pointing to the side. Take a deep inhale.

3. Exhale and turn your torso to the right, holding the position for a few moments.

4. Inhale to return to the center and repeat to the left, doing two reps on each side.

Spinal twists are one of my favorite movements because they can help relieve tension in your spine and improve its flexibility while strengthening your core and posture.

FINISH WITH 2 - 3 MINUTES OF DEEP LATERAL BREATHING Page **15**

ARM SWINGS
10 times in each direction

11

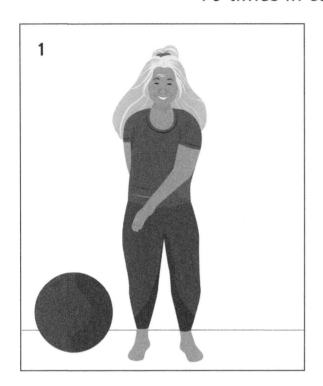

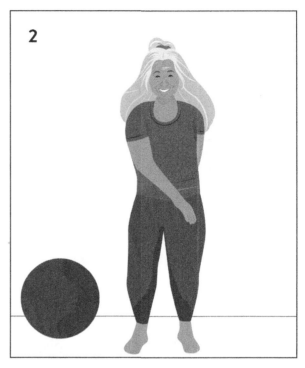

1. Stand with a tall spine and your feet wider than your shoulders. Allow your hands to hang loosely by your side.

2. Turn your torso to the right allowing your arms to swing across and around your body.

3. Turn in the other direction, repeating 10 times each way.

WALL ANGELS
8 to 10 times, 2 sets

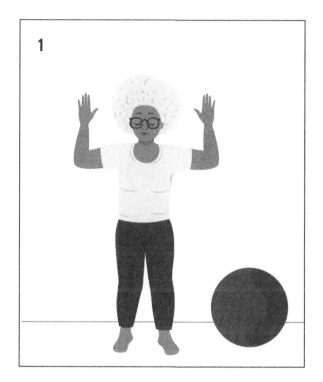 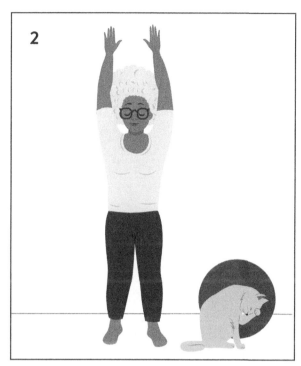

1. Stand about six inches from your wall with your back facing it.

2. Engage your core to straighten your spine.

3. Slightly bend your knees and lean against the wall, ensuring your head, torso, lower back and butt touch it.

4. Lift your arms to a 90 degree angle and open your shoulders. As you move your arms into this position, ensure your arms and elbows stay against the wall.

5. Slide your arms up the wall, keeping your arms and shoulders against the wall, until your hands are as high above your head as you can. Stretch your arms up even further by at least an inch and hold the position for 10 seconds.

6. Still keeping your arms and hands against the wall, slide your arms down until they're back in the starting position (with your elbows at 90 degrees and with your hands at the level of your shoulders). Repeat this 8 - 10 times and do 2 sets.

The point of doing wall angels is to open up your shoulders from the hunched forward position that a lot of us do during the day. The key is to keep your low back and shoulders up against the wall as you move your arms up, and then down. You should feel a stretch in your shoulders where you normally hunch forward.

SEATED ARM CIRCLES
10 times in each direction, 2 sets

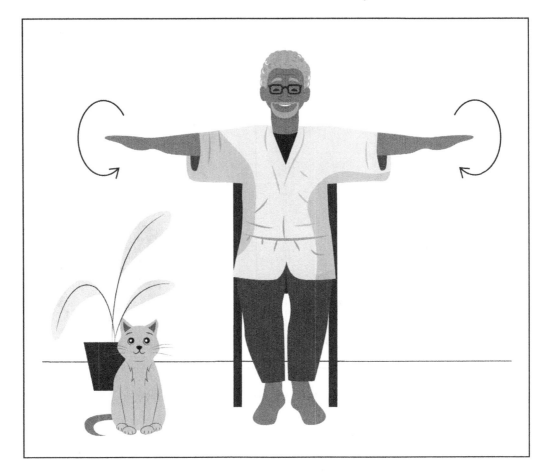

1. Sit in your chair with a lengthened spine. Ensure your core muscles are engaged.

2. Extend your arms to make a "T" shape with your palms facing the floor.

3. Start making small circles from your shoulder joint with your arms circling to the back. Continue doing this, making your circles larger each time for 30 seconds.

4. Lower your arms and shake them out.

5. Lift them back up to the "T" shape and repeat with your circles going to the front for 30 seconds.

6. Repeat 10 times in each direction and do 2 sets.

WEEK TWO - DAY FOUR

SEATED SINGLE-LEG EXTENSION
10 reps on each side, 2 sets

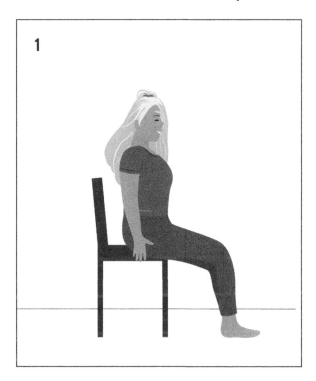
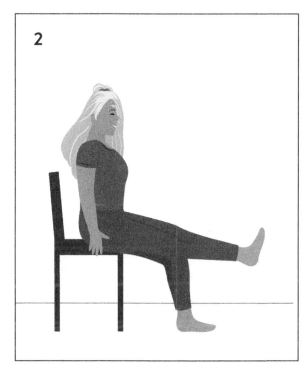

1. Sit near the edge of your seat with your legs hip-width apart.

2. Engage your core to lengthen your spine. Place your hands on either side of the chair seat. Take a deep breath in.

3. Exhale to lift your left leg. Stop when your leg is straight out from your hip. Lower and repeat 10 times.

4. Switch sides. Do 2 sets.

BONUS CHAIR EXERCISE

WEEK TWO - DAY FOUR

SEATED SIDE BEND

15 reps on each side

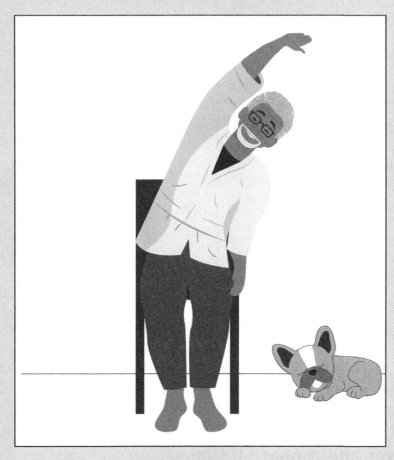

1. Sit in your chair with your feet hip distance apart. Ensure your knees stay stacked over your ankles.

2. Engage your core to lengthen your spine. Pull your shoulders back and away from your ears.

3. Keeping your left hand on your chair's left side, sweep your right arm over your head and lean toward your left to feel a stretch in your right side. Be careful not to twist your torso or lean too forward, backward, or sideways.

4. Switch sides, and continue alternating until you've completed this exercise 15 times on each side.

WEEK TWO - DAY FOUR

WALL-ASSISTED PECTORAL STRETCH
Hold for 20 seconds on each side, 2 sets

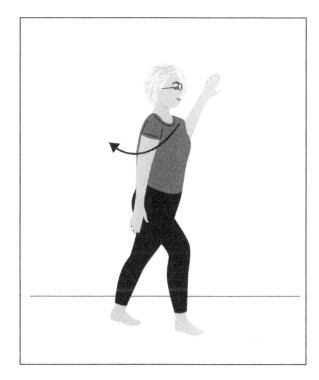

11

1. Stand with your left side facing the wall. Bend your left arm and place your left forearm on the wall, at shoulder height.

2. Step forward with your right leg, and at the same time, slightly rotate your left shoulder forward and out towards the right. It's important that your forearm doesn't move and that all the stretching motion is coming from your left pectoral muscle /left side of your chest.

3. Hold for 20 seconds, then relax. Repeat one more time on the same side.

4. Turn around, switch sides and do the pectoral stretch twice on that side too.

Our chest muscles are prone to becoming tight due to sitting for a long time and hunching over. By using the wall to stretch your chest muscles, you'll be able to loosen the muscles, decrease any pain caused by the tightness, and increase your flexibility and mobility in your upper body.

OVERHEAD WALL CHEST STRETCH
Hold for 20 seconds, 2 sets

11

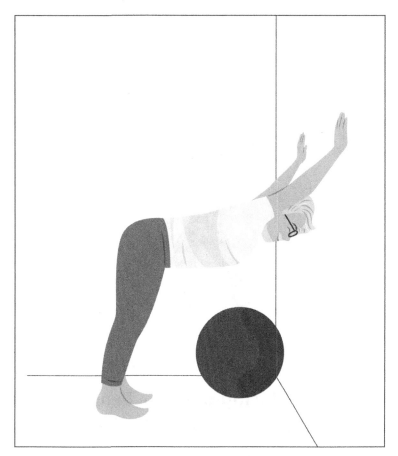

1. **Stand an arm's length away from your wall, facing it.**

2. **Raise your arms above your head. Place your hands against the wall.**

3. **Maintaining your straight arms, lean forward to press your chest against the wall, stopping when you feel a stretch in your upper chest.**

4. **Hold for 20 seconds, then relax and repeat. Do 2 sets.**

FINISH WITH 2 - 3 MINUTES OF DEEP LATERAL BREATHING
Page
15

WEEK TWO - DAY FIVE

BEGIN WITH 1 MINUTE OF DEEP LATERAL BREATHING Page 15

NECK ROLLS
5 times in each direction

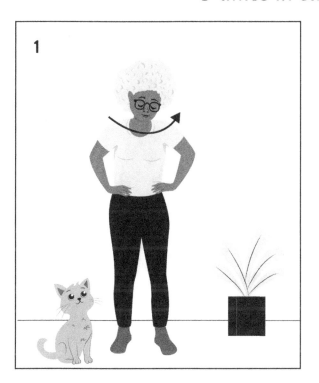

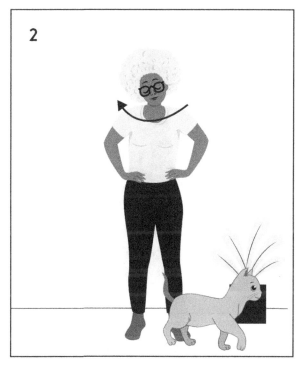

1. Stand tall with your hands on your waist and your head facing forward. Ensure your shoulders are away from your ears and your core supports your posture.

2. Tuck your chin down towards your neck and slowly roll your head to the left, until your chin is above your left shoulder, and you're looking slightly upwards and behind you.

3. Drop your chin, and tuck it in as you slowly roll your head down and to the right, until your chin is above your right shoulder, and you're looking slightly upwards and behind you on the right side.

4. Repeat in alternating directions 5 times.

WEEK TWO - DAY FIVE

SHOULDER BLADE SQUEEZES
10 - 20 times

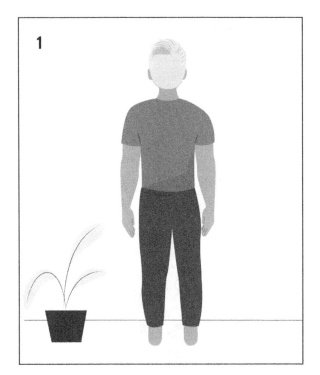 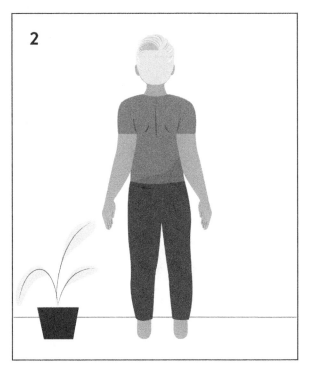

1. Stand with a tall spine, feet about hip-width apart, and arms hanging by your sides.

2. Imagine a lemon between your shoulder blades as you pull your arms and elbows back to squeeze your shoulder blades together.

3. Release and repeat up to 20 times.

Our shoulders are one of the most important joints in our upper body, however these joints are used too often, especially when lifting. Shoulder blade squeezes help maintain your joints' stability and improve your posture.

STANDING WALL CRUNCHES
10 times, 1 or 2 sets

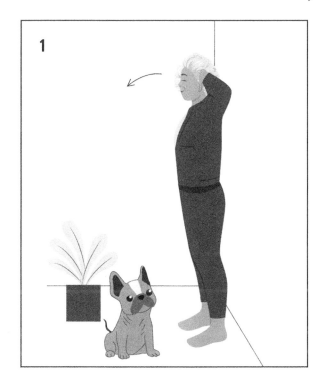 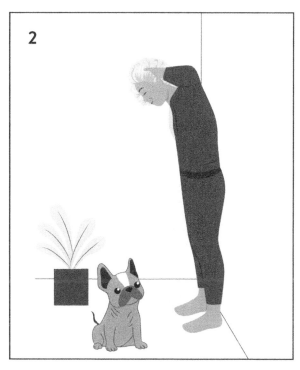

12

1. Stand about six to eight inches from your wall with your legs hip-width apart. Rest your hips, mid and upper back, and your head against the wall, ensuring your lower back and neck are not touching it. Place your hands against the back of your head.

2. Engage your abs and fold forward, starting with your upper back. Continue to bend at your waist as you push your ribs back to have your lower back touch the wall. Ensure you are breathing out as you contract your abs.

3. Inhale to return to the starting position. Repeat the crunch until you have completed between 10 and 20 reps.

Traditional crunches help build muscles in your abdominal region to improve your core's stability and protect your back from injury—but they can cause discomfort in your back or neck when performing them, which is why standing crunches are ideal.

WEEK TWO - DAY FIVE

WALL PUSH-UPS
5 - 10 times

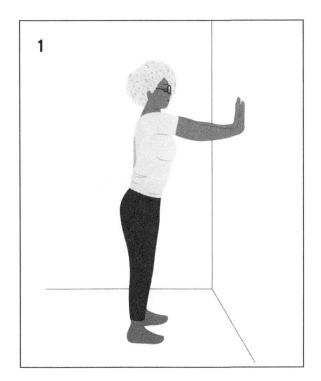 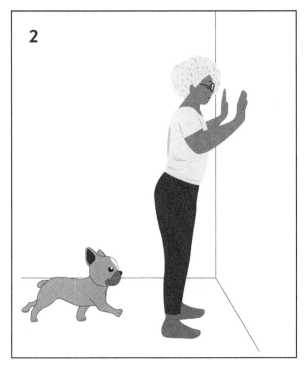

12

1. Stand no more than two feet from the wall, adjusting the distance according to your fitness level. You'll want to be closer to the wall if traditional push-ups are hard for you.

2. Place your hands on the wall at your shoulder height, just a bit wider than your shoulder width, and fingers are pointing up to the ceiling. Adjust your legs to be hip-width apart.

3. Engage your core and inhale.

4. Exhale to lower your chest toward the wall.

5. Inhale to push back up to the start and repeat.

6. Continue until you have completed 5 - 10 push-ups.

WALL-ASSISTED CROSS-BODY SHOULDER STRETCH
Holding for 20 seconds, 5 sets on each side

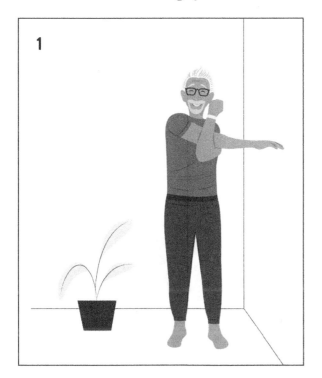 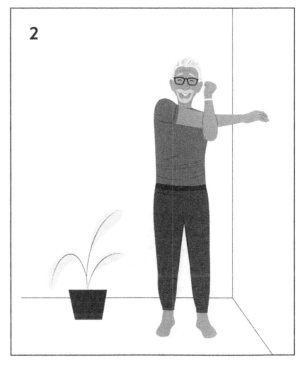

12

1. Stand about an arm's distance from your wall with your left side facing it.

2. Bring your right arm across your chest, keeping it straight, and place your hand against the wall for support.

3. Using your left hand, press against your right shoulder until you feel a stretch in your upper back and right shoulder.

4. Hold for 20 seconds, then switch to your left arm. Do it 5 sets.

WALL SHOULDER EXTENSION STRETCH
Hold for 20 seconds, 2 sets

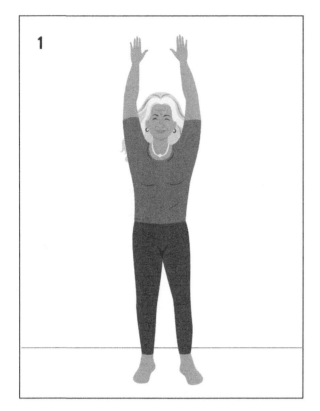
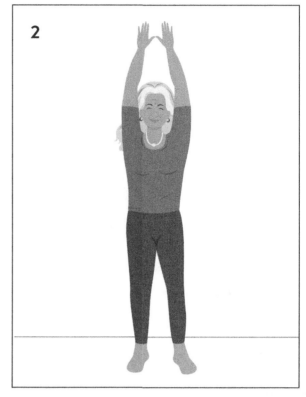

1. Stand with your feet shoulder-width apart and your back against the wall.

2. Extend your arms above your head with the backs of your hands resting against the wall.

3. Keeping your elbows straight, slide your hands up the wall until you feel a stretch in your shoulders.

4. Hold for 20 seconds. Do 2 sets.

FINISH WITH 2 - 3 MINUTES OF DEEP LATERAL BREATHING Page **15**

BEGIN WITH 1 MINUTE OF DEEP LATERAL BREATHING Page 15

SEATED ARM CIRCLES
10 times in each direction, 2 sets

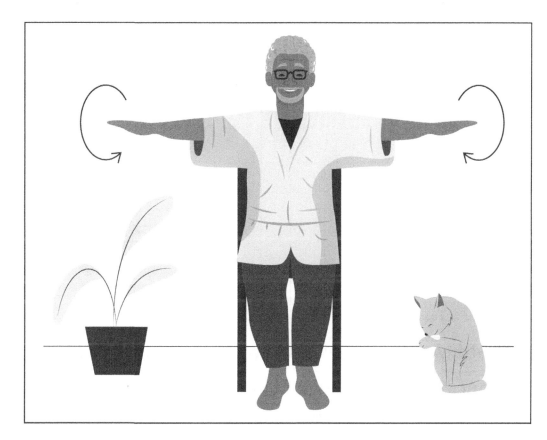

13

1. Sit in your chair with a lengthened spine. Ensure your core muscles are engaged.

2. Extend your arms to make a "T" shape with your palms facing the floor.

3. Start making small circles from your shoulder joint with your arms circling to the back. Continue doing this, making your circles larger each time for 30 seconds.

4. Lower your arms and shake them out.

5. Lift them back up to the "T" shape and repeat with your circles going to the front for 30 seconds.

6. Repeat 10 times in each direction and do 2 sets.

TORSO TWISTS
1 minute

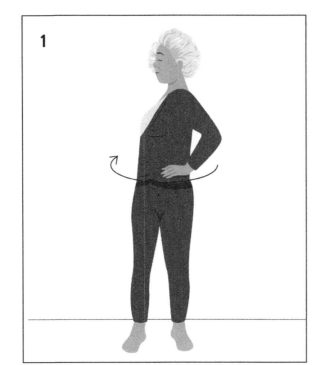 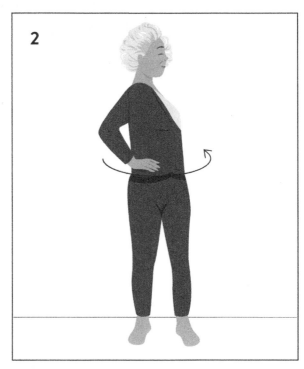

1. Stand tall with your feet hip-width apart and your hands on your waist.

2. Keeping your feet planted, twist your torso to the right as far as you can go, then twist the other way. Engage your core muscles and keep your feet planted on the floor so that the stretch is focused on your torso.

3. Repeat 5 to 10 times in each direction, or do more for up to a full minute.

WEEK TWO - DAY SIX

TRADITIONAL WALL PLANK
Hold for 10 - 30 seconds

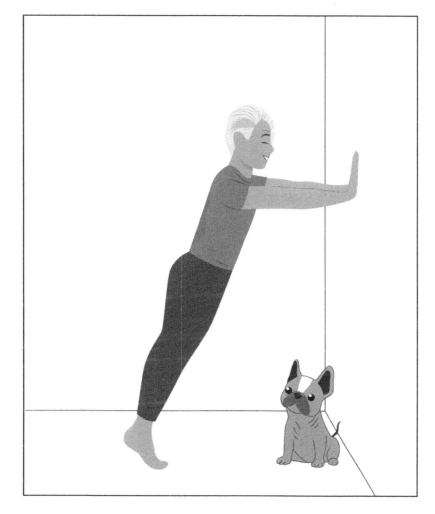

1. **Start with your hands resting against the wall, your arms straight, and your legs hip-width apart and slightly back from the wall to put your body in a straight diagonal.**
   To make this exercise more challenging, then instead of having your arms straight, bend them and rest your forearms against the wall.

2. **Engage your core and try to hold for as long as possible, but aim for at least 10 seconds and work up from there.**

Planks have plenty of benefits, especially for strengthening your core muscles. Using the wall will provide you with more stabilization for your core while helping you find a better balance.

ADVANCED EXERCISE

WEEK TWO - DAY SIX

SIDE PLANK WITH ROTATION
2 -3 times on each side

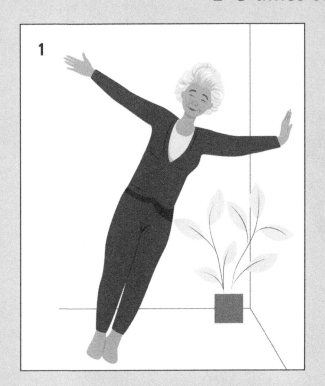

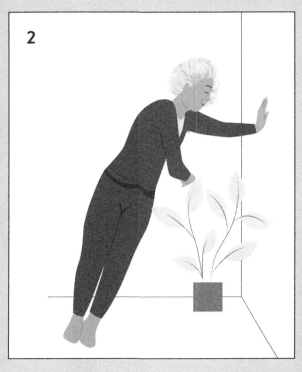

1. Start in the side plank position against the wall, leaning against your left arm.

2. Extend your right arm beside you to make half of a "T" shape.

3. Move your right arm down and under your upper body as if you're going to hug your belly.

4. Untwist to return to the starting position, extend your arm beside you, then repeat 10 times on each side.

ADVANCED EXERCISE

WEEK TWO - DAY SIX

MCCONNELL SQUAT
5 - 10 times

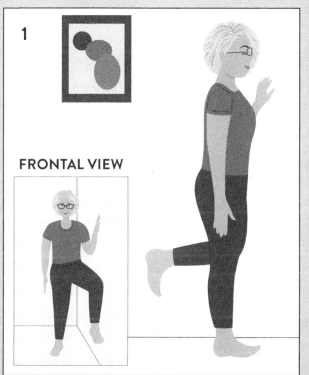

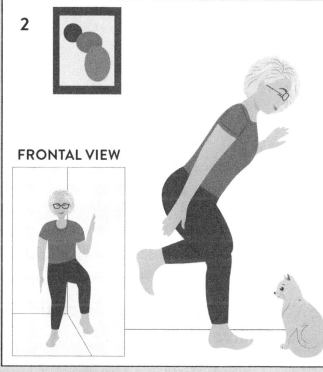

1. Stand with your left side facing the wall, and with your left hand resting against it.

2. Lift your left leg, with your left knee at a 90 degree angle, and push the side of your calf and thigh into the wall. That's right, you have your left hand on the wall and you're pushing the side of your left leg into the wall as well. This is so you have proper support for the next move.

3. Push your hand and the side of your leg into the wall for support, while you bend your right knee and simultaneously squat down with your butt, as far as you comfortable can.

4. Hold the squat for 10 seconds, then stand back up. Repeat 5 -10 times (or as many as you can), and then switch sides and legs.

The McConnell squat is one of the most difficult in this book. That said, it's an excellent one-legged Pilates exercise for improving your balance, flexibility, stability and for reducing back pain by strengthening your quads, hamstrings, glutes, and core muscles! If you're not up to it, then skip for now, but when you're ready for the challenge, it's worth it!

WEEK TWO - DAY SIX

SEATED SPINAL TWISTS
2 times on each side

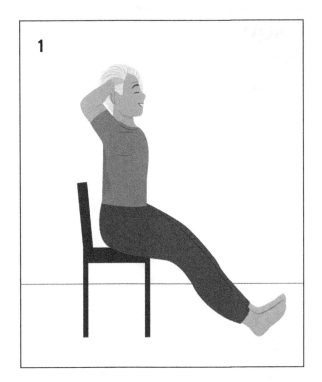 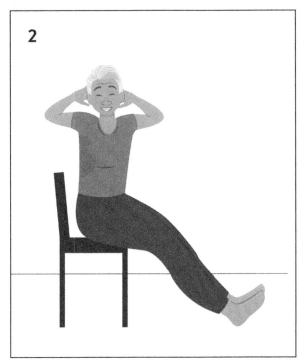

1. Sit in the center of your chair. Engage your core to lengthen your spine. Have your legs slightly wider than your hips.

2. Place your hands on the back of your head with your elbows pointing to the side. Take a deep inhale.

3. Exhale and turn your torso to the right, holding the position for a few moments.

4. Inhale to return to the center and repeat to the left, doing two reps on each side.

Spinal twists are one of my favorite movements because they can help relieve tension in your spine and improve its flexibility while strengthening your core and posture.

SEATED ROLL-DOWN
5 times

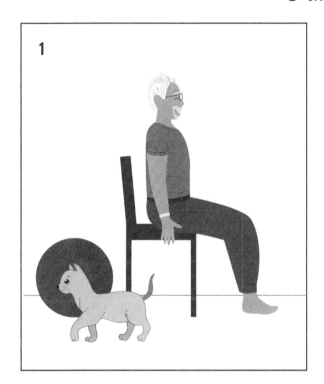

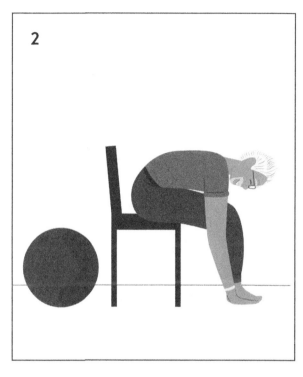

1. Sit near the edge of your seat and rest your hands at your side. Ensure your legs are about hip-width apart.

2. Inhale to engage your core muscles and lengthen your spine.

3. Exhale and slowly roll down, starting with tucking your chin into your chest to round your back and slowly roll down. Allow your hands to dangle in front of you or touch the floor when you are as far as you can go.

4. Hang out for as long as you need. When you are ready, inhale to slowly come back up, picturing your vertebrae stacking on one another as you go.

FINISH WITH 2 - 3 MINUTES OF DEEP LATERAL BREATHING Page 15

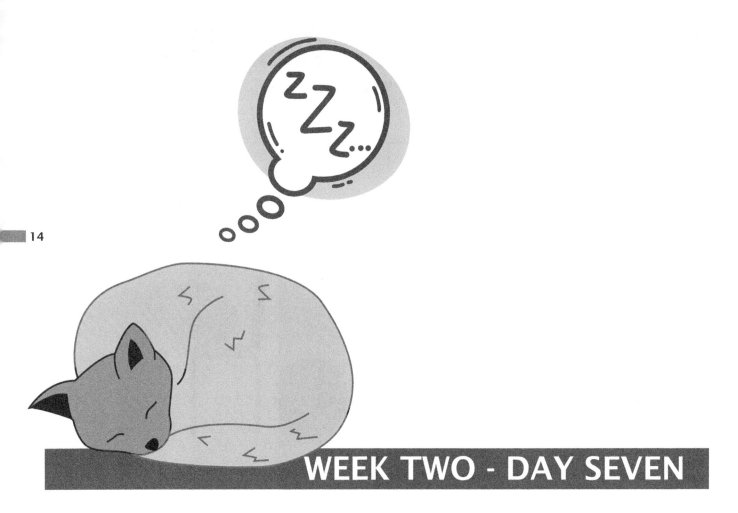

WEEK TWO - DAY SEVEN

REST DAY

BEGIN WITH 1 MINUTE OF DEEP LATERAL BREATHING Page 15

NECK ROLLS
5 times in each direction

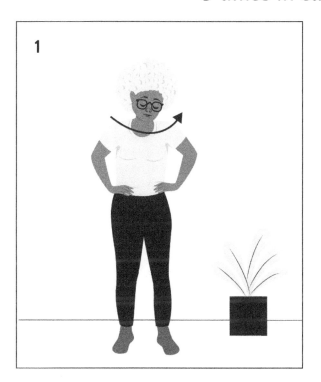

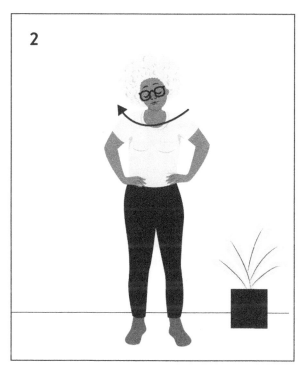

15

1. Stand tall with your hands on your waist and your head facing forward. Ensure your shoulders are away from your ears and your core supports your posture.

2. Tuck your chin down towards your neck and slowly roll your head to the left, until your chin is above your left shoulder, and you're looking slightly upwards and behind you.

3. Drop your chin, and tuck it in as you slowly roll your head down and to the right, until your chin is above your right shoulder, and you're looking slightly upwards and behind you on the right side.

4. Repeat in alternating directions 5 times.

ANKLE PUMPS
10 times with each ankle

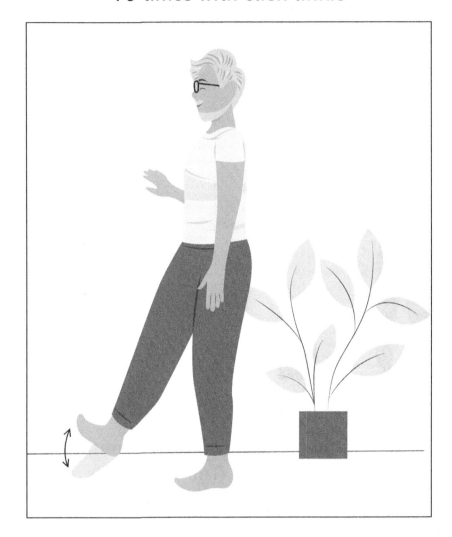

15

1. **Stand tall next to your wall with your right hand resting against it for support.**

2. **Extend your right leg with your heel a few inches above the floor.**

3. **Push your toes down (like you would on a gas pedal), hold for a few seconds, then bring your toes back up and toward your shin.**

4. **Repeat 10 times, then switch legs.**

Ankle pumps help to strengthen the ligaments and tendons in your joints. This exercise will also increase circulation to the area and your ankle's range of motion.

WEEK THREE - DAY ONE

STANDING BICYCLE CRUNCHES
10 - 20 reps

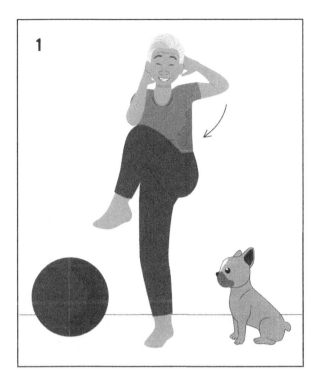 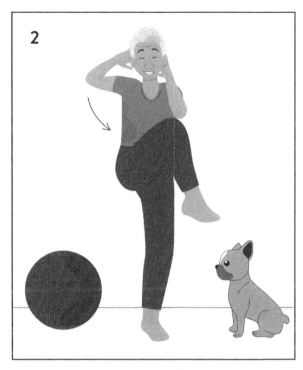

1. **Stand about six to eight inches from your wall with your legs hip-width apart. Rest your hips, mid and upper back, and your head against the wall, ensuring your lower back and neck are not touching it. Place your hands against the back of your head.**

2. **Contract your side abdominal muscles and core, as you twist your midsection to bring your left knee to your right elbow.**

3. **Switch sides.**

4. **Repeat until you have completed between 10 and 20 reps.**

Bicycle crunches are great for targeting your oblique muscles, which are necessary for our stability.

WALL LUNGES
8 to 10 times on each side

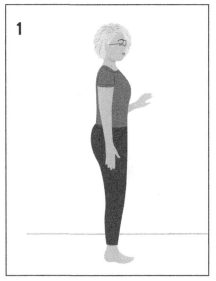 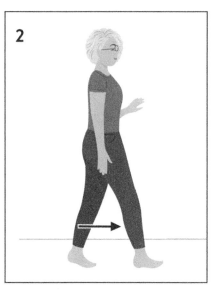 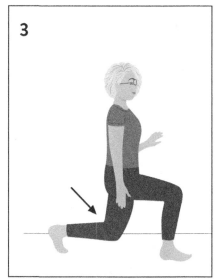

1. Stand with your left side facing the wall and rest your hand on it for support. Ensure your shoulders are back and away from your ears, and you lean forward slightly.

2. Engage your core and step back with your left leg while bending your left knee to about 90 degrees.

3. Press into your right leg to come back to standing.

4. Continue until you have completed between 8 and 10 reps, then switch legs.

Lunges, in general, are great for strengthening our knees because they work your glutes and quads.

NOTE: If this is too hard or causes any knee pain, consider doing a Reverse Lunge on p.51.

WALL-ASSISTED QUAD STRETCH
Holding 30 seconds on each leg, 3 sets

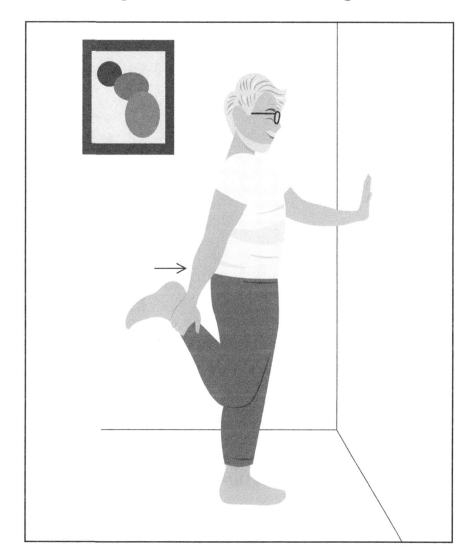

15

1. Stand with your left hand against your wall.

2. Bend your right knee and grab your ankle with your right hand. Bring your heel as close to your bottom as possible until you feel a stretch in the front of your thigh.

3. Hold for 30 seconds.

4. Release, then switch legs. Do 3 sets.

WALL-ASSISTED HAMSTRING STRETCH
Holding 20 seconds on each leg, at least 3 times

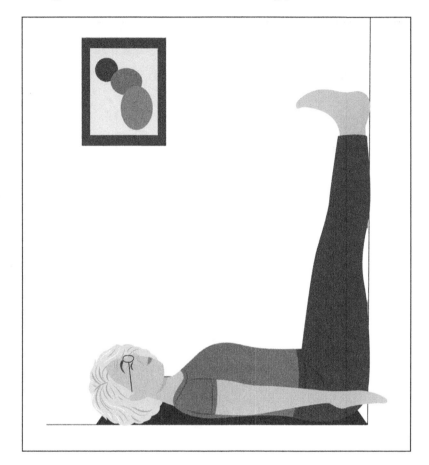

15

1. Lie in front of your wall with your legs resting against it, extended upwards toward the ceiling.

2. Shimmy your bottom close to the wall.

3. Press your heels into the wall as you straighten your knee until you feel a stretch in your hamstrings.

4. Hold for 20 seconds, then relax. Repeat at least 3 times or more if you can.

NOTE: This is one of the few exercises that's on the floor. If you don't feel comfortable, then try the Wall Roll Down on p.61 or the Seated Heel Slides on p.107 as a alternate hamstring stretch.

FINISH WITH 2 - 3 MINUTES OF DEEP LATERAL BREATHING
Page
15

BEGIN WITH 1 MINUTE OF DEEP LATERAL BREATHING Page 15

SHOULDER ROLLS
10 times in each direction

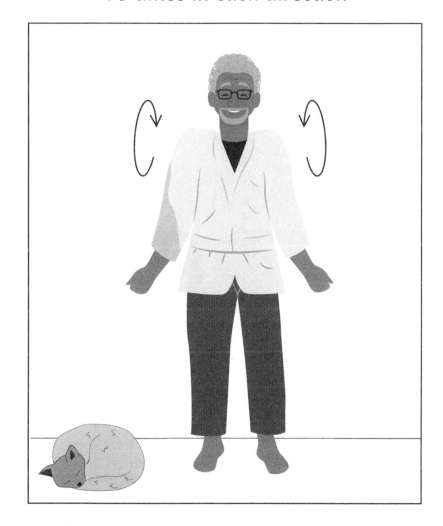

16

1. **Stand with a tall spine and your feet about hip-width apart. Allow your hands to dangle by your sides.**

2. **Begin rolling your shoulders backward by lifting them toward your ears and then back. Continue until you have completed 10 rotations.**

3. **To roll your shoulders forward, you will begin by squeezing your shoulder blades and then lifting your shoulders toward your ears. Push your shoulders forward, then back down. Continue until you have completed 10 rotations.**

ARM SWINGS
10 times in each direction

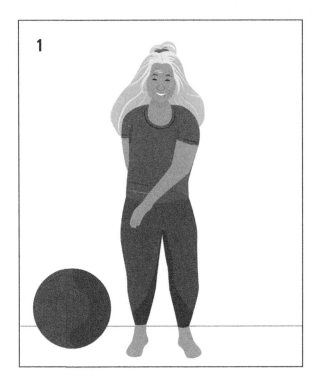
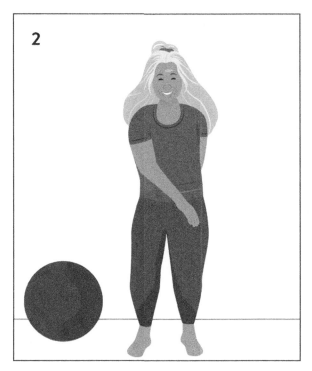

16

1. Stand with a tall spine and your feet wider than your shoulders. Allow your hands to hang loosely by your side.

2. Turn your torso to the right allowing your arms to swing across and around your body.

3. Turn in the other direction, repeating 10 times each way.

WALL SLIDES WITH EXTERNAL ROTATION
15 to 20 times, 2 sets

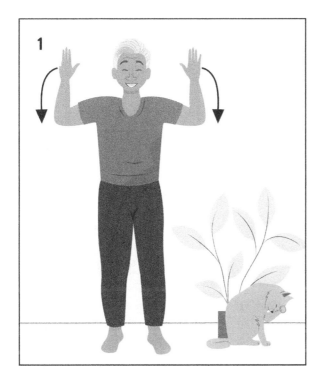 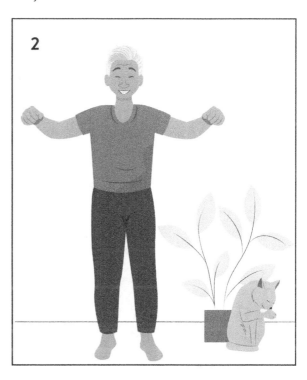

16

1. Stand with your back facing the wall, and with your feet about a foot away from the wall.

2. Put your hips and shoulders up against the wall, making sure that you don't arch your back too far away from the wall, and tuck your stomach in. Keep your elbows and forearms against the wall.

3. In a controlled manner, slowly rotate your forearms forward in a downward motion towards the floor. Keep your wrists in line with your forearms.

4. Stop when your forearms are at a 90 degree angle (basically at your natural shoulder / upper chest height). Then rotate your forearms back up, keeping your wrists inline, until your forearms are up against the wall again. Repeat. Do 2 sets of 15 - 20 times.

You should feel this in exercise in the back of your shoulders, and right at the join of your arm to your armpit. It's a fantastic exercise to increase the flexibility in your shoulders, which will give you better posture with your shoulders held back!

WALL SQUAT WITH (OR WITHOUT) A STABILITY BALL
8 to 10 reps, 2 sets

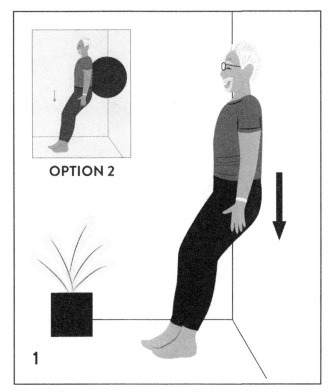

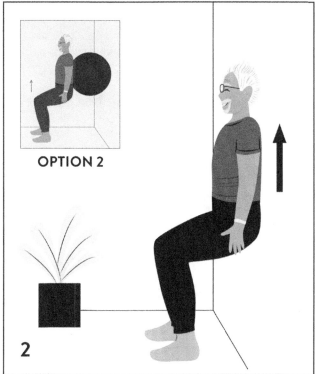

1. **If using the ball, place the ball between the curve of your lower back and the wall, resting your back on the ball. If you're not using the ball, simply rest your back on the wall itself.**

2. **Take a small step forward (about six inches).**

3. **Engage your core and inhale.**

4. **Exhale as you lower yourself, stopping when your knees are at a 90-degree angle.**

5. **Inhale as you stand back up.**

6. **Do 2 sets of 8 to 10 reps.**

If you are not feeling strong enough to execute a squat, a stability ball will be your new best friend. A stability ball can help you find proper form while supporting you through the movement. When choosing a stability ball, it's good to select one for your height. For example, if you're between 5' and 5'5", you'll want to select a ball that is 2 feet in diameter.

BONUS CHAIR EXERCISE

WEEK THREE - DAY TWO

SEATED HEEL SLIDES
10 reps

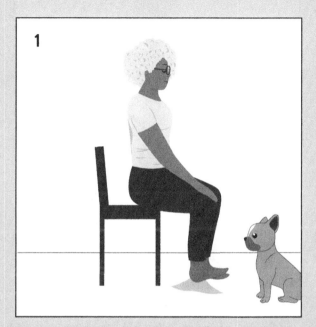 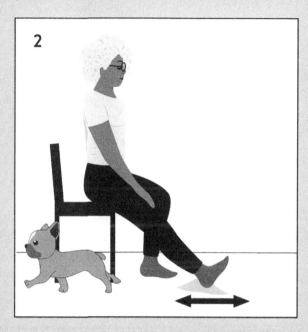

1. Sit in your chair, facing forward with your legs hip-width apart. Place a tea towel under your right heel (or a piece of paper if you're on a carpeted floor) and flex your ankle to have your toes pointed to the ceiling.

2. Press into your heel and push the tea towel out to extend your leg.

3. Press into the tea towel as you activate your hamstrings to bring the towel back.

4. Repeat 10 times.

Heel slides focus on activating your hamstrings to balance out the work your quad muscles do daily. This can help protect your knee from an injury while increasing circulation to your knee joint. This is especially important if you have an arthritic knee.

You'll need a non-carpeted floor and a folded tea towel for this exercise. Alternatively, fitness sliders are available, and these dual-sided discs can slide on a carpet or hardwood flooring.

FORWARD BEND

1 time

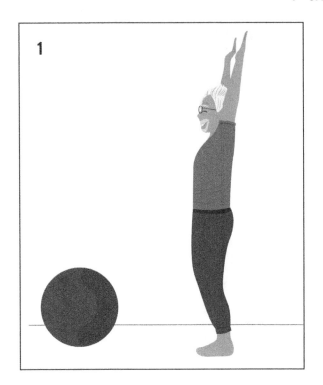
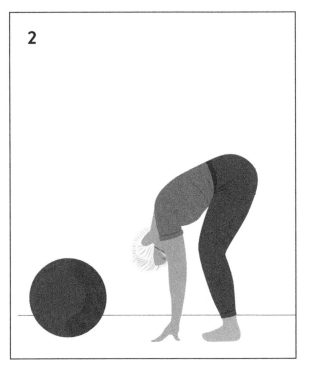

1. Stand with a straight spine and your feet about hip distance apart.

2. Reach your arms up overhead, then lower your arms down on both of your sides as you hinge at your hips to fold forward.

3. Aim to touch the floor if you can, but don't push yourself past what your body can comfortably do. Allow your head to hang as you breathe into the stretch.

4. Place your hands on your thighs or hips, and engage your core muscles to roll back up slowly one vertebrae at a time.

SEATED ROLL-DOWN

5 times

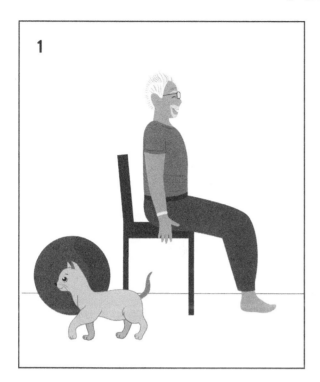

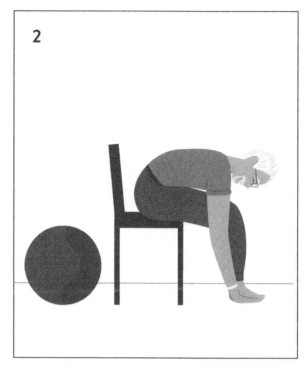

16

1. Sit near the edge of your seat and rest your hands at your side. Ensure your legs are about hip-width apart.

2. Inhale to engage your core muscles and lengthen your spine.

3. Exhale and slowly roll down, starting with tucking your chin into your chest to round your back and slowly roll down. Allow your hands to dangle in front of you or touch the floor when you are as far as you can go.

4. Hang out for as long as you need. When you are ready, inhale to slowly come back up, picturing your vertebrae stacking on one another as you go.

FINISH WITH 2 - 3 MINUTES OF DEEP LATERAL BREATHING Page **15**

BEGIN WITH 1 MINUTE OF DEEP LATERAL BREATHING Page 15

TORSO TWISTS
1 minute

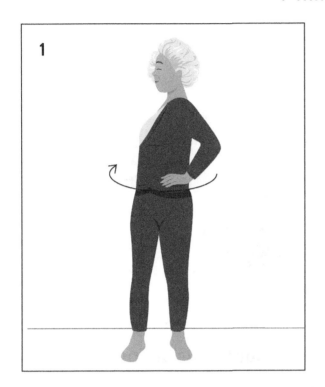

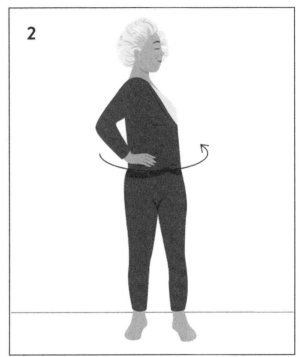

1. Stand tall with your feet hip-width apart and your hands on your waist.

2. Keeping your feet planted, twist your torso to the right as far as you can go, then twist the other way. Engage your core muscles and keep your feet planted on the floor so that the stretch is focused on your torso.

3. Repeat 5 to 10 times in each direction, or do more for up to a full minute.

WEEK THREE - DAY THREE

STANDING SIDE BRIDGE WALL SLIDES
15 to 20 times on each side, 2 sets

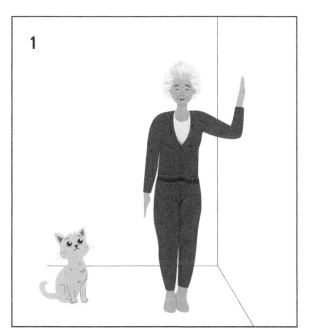 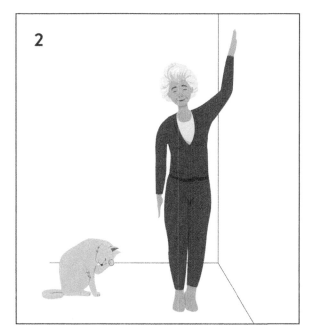

1. Stand with your left side facing the wall, with a small space between your feet.

2. Bend your left elbow and lean your forearm against the wall, at shoulder height.

3. Engage your core and slide your left arm slowly, straight up the wall. Your natural tendency will be to drop your right shoulder and lean your head and shoulders to the right. This is good, but you want to keep your body in line. To help this, point the fingers of your right hand down towards the floor and allow the right side of your body to lean away from the wall, while your left hand and arm slowly move up the wall. Keep your shoulders, neck and head in line with each other..

4. You're creating a slight 'bridge' as your body does a standing curve.

5. The movement is subtle and controlled. This exercise helps your posture, as you focus on keeping your head, neck and shoulders in line, while the sides of your abdomen make the slight curve up and away from the wall.

6. Repeat 15 - 20 times on each side. Do 2 sets.

TRADITIONAL WALL PLANK
Hold for 10 - 30 seconds

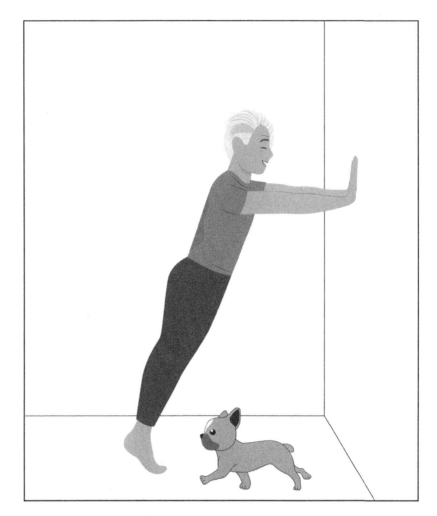

17

1. **Start with your hands resting against the wall, your arms straight, and your legs hip-width apart and slightly back from the wall to put your body in a straight diagonal.**
   To make this exercise more challenging, then instead of having your arms straight, bend them and rest your forearms against the wall.

2. **Engage your core and try to hold for as long as possible, but aim for at least 10 seconds and work up from there.**

Planks have plenty of benefits, especially for strengthening your core muscles. Using the wall will provide you with more stabilization for your core while helping you find a better balance.

BONUS EXERCISE

WEEK THREE - DAY THREE

ONE-ARM WALL PLANK
Hold for 10 - 30 seconds on each side

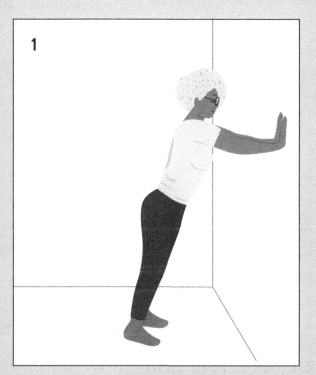 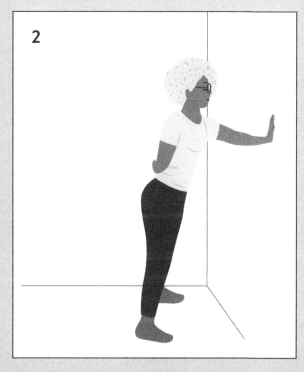

1. Start with your hands resting against the wall, your arms straight, and your legs hip-width apart and slightly back from the wall to put your body in a straight diagonal.

2. Lift your right hand from the wall and put it behind your back. If you want to challenge yourself a little more, then hold your right arm out to the side (so that you're making half of a "T" shape).

3. Keep your core engaged to ensure your body remains straight, aiming to hold the position for 10 seconds and work up from there.

4. Return your right hand to the wall and relax.

5. Repeat the same steps with your left arm off the wall.

FORWARD BEND

1 time

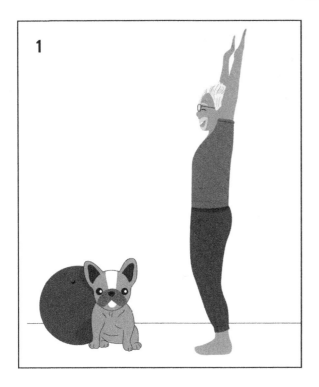
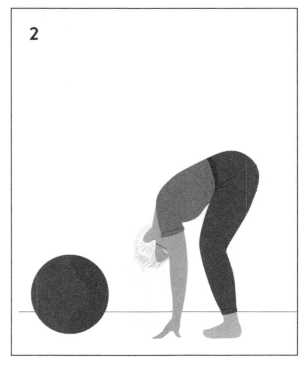

1. Stand with a straight spine and your feet about hip distance apart.

2. Reach your arms up overhead, then lower your arms down on both of your sides as you hinge at your hips to fold forward.

3. Aim to touch the floor if you can, but don't push yourself past what your body can comfortably do. Allow your head to hang as you breathe into the stretch.

4. Place your hands on your thighs or hips, and engage your core muscles to roll back up slowly one vertebrae at a time.

WEEK THREE - DAY THREE

CAT-COWS
5 times

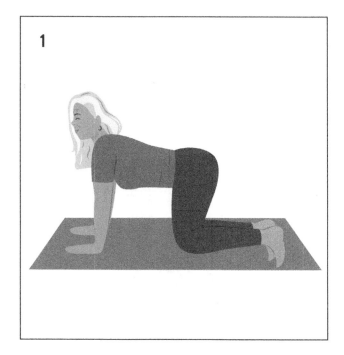

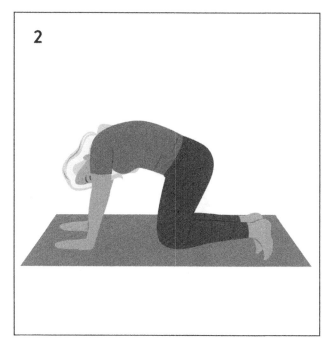

1. Get on your hands and knees on your mat in a tabletop position. Ensure your hips are stacked over your knees, and your shoulders are over your wrists.

2. Engage your core to keep your spine straight.

3. Breathe in as you tilt your pelvis and look up to the ceiling to create a "C" shape. This is your cow position.

4. Exhale and round your back as you round your spine and tuck your tailbone in, creating a scaredy-cat arch.

5. Repeat 5 times.

NOTE: This is one of the few exercises that's on the floor. If you don't feel comfortable, then repeat the Forward Bend from the previous page, and curl your back into more of an arch once your hands are on the floor.

FINISH WITH 2 - 3 MINUTES OF DEEP LATERAL BREATHING Page 15

LEG SWINGS
10 times with each leg

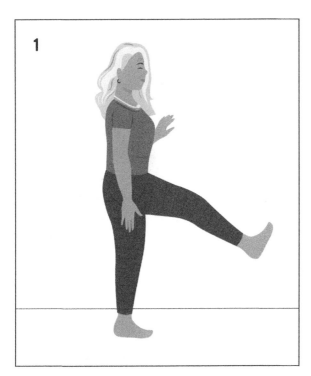

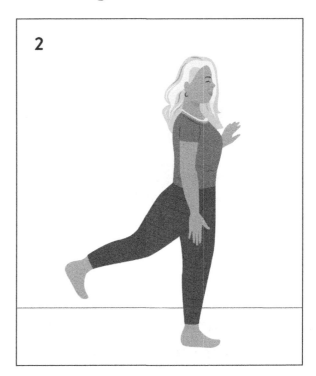

1. **Stand with your left side facing your wall. Engage your core muscles to keep you from losing your balance.**

2. **Keeping your left leg stationary, begin swinging your right leg forward and backward, aiming to swing higher each time.**

3. **Repeat 10 times in each direction, then switch sides.**

If you spend a significant amount of time sitting, it will impact your hip flexors because they become compressed. Over time, it can lead to pain and mobility issues. However, leg swings can help warm up and stretch the muscles and tendons in your hip joint, relieving any discomfort and removing your hips from a compressed position.

ANKLE PUMPS
10 times with each ankle

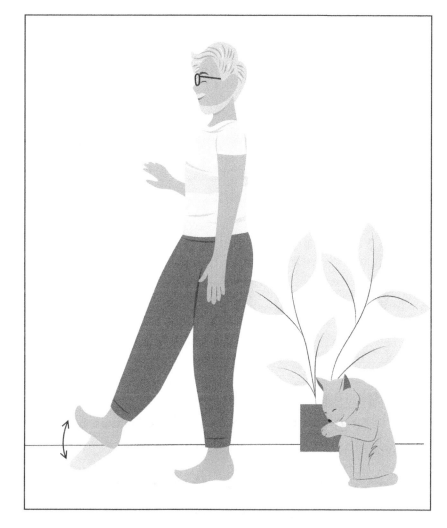

18

1. **Stand tall next to your wall with your right hand resting against it for support.**

2. **Extend your right leg with your heel a few inches above the floor.**

3. **Push your toes down (like you would on a gas pedal), hold for a few seconds, then bring your toes back up and toward your shin.**

4. **Repeat 10 times, then switch legs.**

Ankle pumps help to strengthen the ligaments and tendons in your joints. This exercise will also increase circulation to the area and your ankle's range of motion.

MARCHING
1 minute

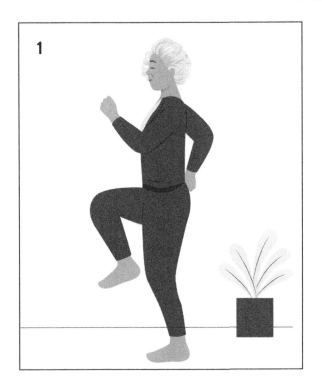 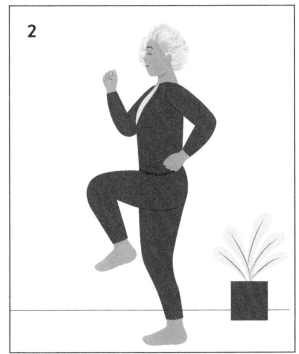

1. Stand on your yoga mat with your feet hip-width apart. Engage your core muscles to straighten your spine. Your feet should be facing the front.

2. Lift your right leg as high as possible while simultaneously lifting your left arm with a bent elbow. Lower your leg and arm and repeat on the other side with your opposite arm and leg.

3. Continue alternating your legs until you've completed 12 to 15 on each side, or do up to 1 minute.

Get a boost of cardio with this warm-up exercise! Marching will help to boost your heart rate and increase the mobility and flexibility in your hips and quadriceps.

SEATED SCISSOR LEGS
15 times

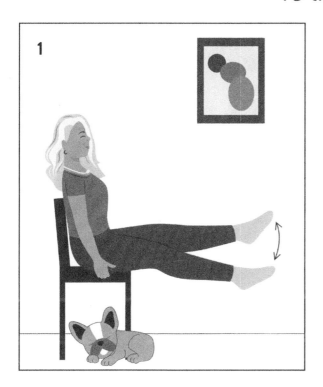 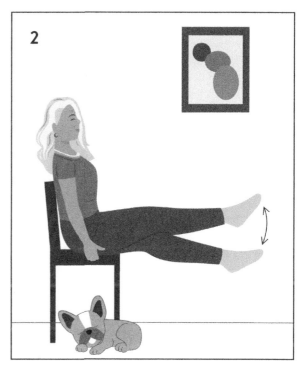

1. Sit in your chair with your bottom slightly forward from the middle. Support yourself by placing your hands on either side of your chair seat.

2. Lift your legs straight in front of you, keeping your ankles slightly relaxed.

3. Engage your core muscles to lengthen your spine.

4. Cross your right leg over the left, then switch, continuing to alternate between legs. Ensure that as you scissor your legs, your shoulders are not creeping up to your ears.

5. Continue the exercise for up to one minute.

SEATED SIDE BEND
15 reps on each side

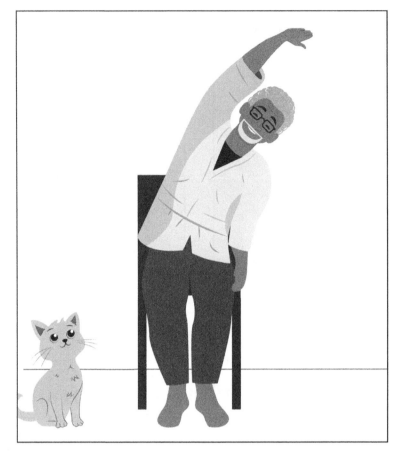

1. Sit in your chair with your feet hip distance apart. Ensure your knees stay stacked over your ankles.

2. Engage your core to lengthen your spine. Pull your shoulders back and away from your ears.

3. Keeping your left hand on your chair's left side, sweep your right arm over your head and lean toward your left to feel a stretch in your right side. Be careful not to twist your torso or lean too forward, backward, or sideways.

4. Switch sides, and continue alternating until you've completed this exercise 15 times on each side.

SEATED HIP FLEXOR STRETCH

Holding for 20 seconds, 2 sets

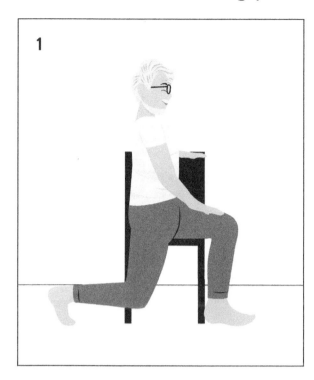 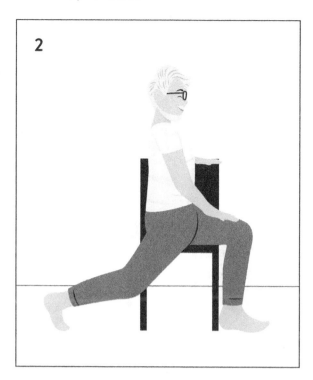

1. Sit sideways in your chair with your left side facing the backrest.

2. Extend your right leg as far behind you as possible until you feel a stretch in your hip and thigh. The ball of your foot should be placed flat on the floor, and your heel should be lifted. Ensure your spine is tall by engaging your core muscles.

3. Hold for 20 seconds.

4. Bring your leg back in, then switch sides. Do 2 sets.

SEATED ROLL-DOWN
5 times

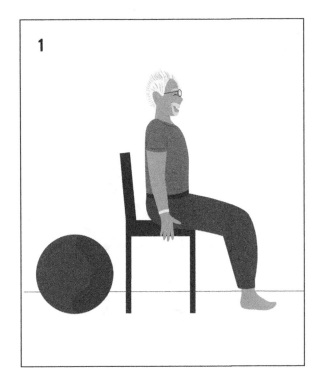

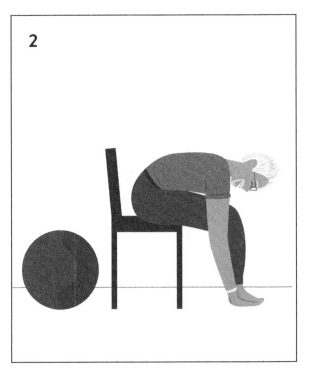

18

1. Sit near the edge of your seat and rest your hands at your side. Ensure your legs are about hip-width apart.

2. Inhale to engage your core muscles and lengthen your spine.

3. Exhale and slowly roll down, starting with tucking your chin into your chest to round your back and slowly roll down. Allow your hands to dangle in front of you or touch the floor when you are as far as you can go.

4. Hang out for as long as you need. When you are ready, inhale to slowly come back up, picturing your vertebrae stacking on one another as you go.

FINISH WITH 2 - 3 MINUTES OF DEEP LATERAL BREATHING Page **15**

WEEK THREE - DAY FIVE

BEGIN WITH 1 MINUTE OF DEEP LATERAL BREATHING Page **15**

SEATED ARM CIRCLES
10 times in each direction, 2 sets

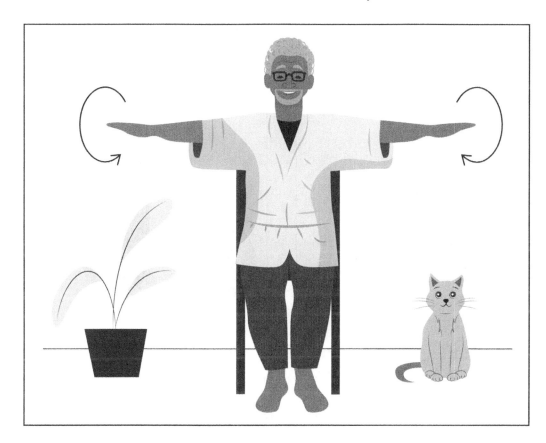

19

1. Sit in your chair with a lengthened spine. Ensure your core muscles are engaged.

2. Extend your arms to make a "T" shape with your palms facing the floor.

3. Start making small circles from your shoulder joint with your arms circling to the back. Continue doing this, making your circles larger each time for 30 seconds.

4. Lower your arms and shake them out.

5. Lift them back up to the "T" shape and repeat with your circles going to the front for 30 seconds.

6. Repeat 10 times in each direction and do 2 sets.

ARM SWINGS
10 times in each direction

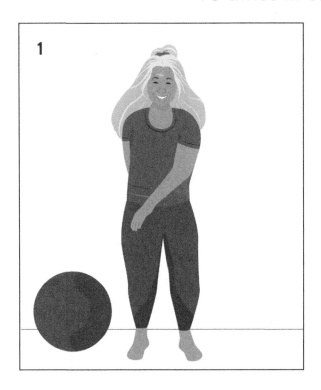 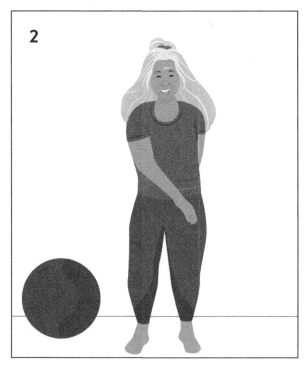

1. Stand with a tall spine and your feet wider than your shoulders. Allow your hands to hang loosely by your side.

2. Turn your torso to the right allowing your arms to swing across and around your body.

3. Turn in the other direction, repeating 10 times each way.

BOXING PUNCHES

10 to 20 times on each side (or 1 minute)

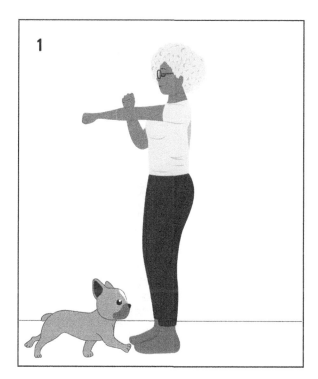 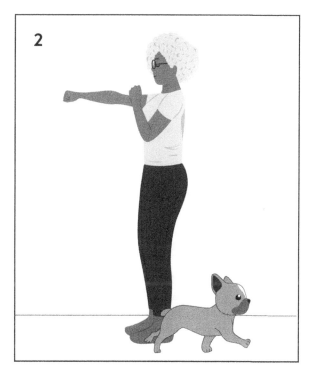

1. Stand with your feet about hip-width apart. Ensure your shoulders are down and away from your ears. Close your hands to make fists, bringing your arms in front of you like a boxer.

2. Punch your left arm out in front of you, then bring it back. Switch sides.

3. Repeat 10 to 20 times, or up to 1 minute.

Boxing punches are a cardio movement to help increase the circulation in your arms and even though you feel you're not moving too much, your heart rate will increase.

WALL PUSH-UPS
5 - 10 times

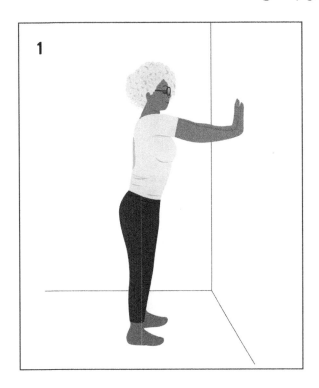 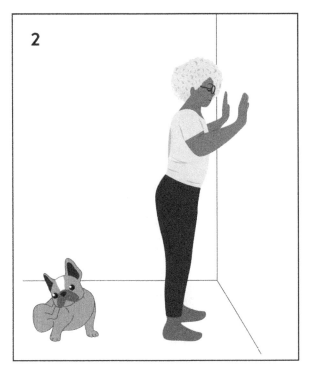

1. Stand no more than two feet from the wall, adjusting the distance according to your fitness level. You'll want to be closer to the wall if traditional push-ups are hard for you.

2. Place your hands on the wall at your shoulder height, just a bit wider than your shoulder width, and fingers are pointing up to the ceiling. Adjust your legs to be hip-width apart.

3. Engage your core and inhale.

4. Exhale to lower your chest toward the wall.

5. Inhale to push back up to the start and repeat.

6. Continue until you have completed 5 - 10 push-ups.

BONUS EXERCISE

WEEK THREE - DAY FIVE

STAGGERED WALL PUSH-UPS

3 - 5 reps on each side

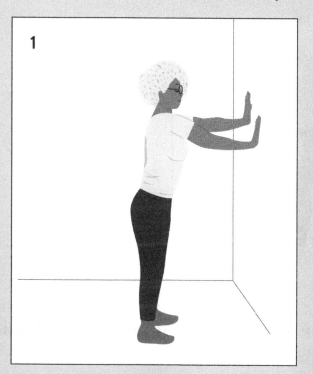 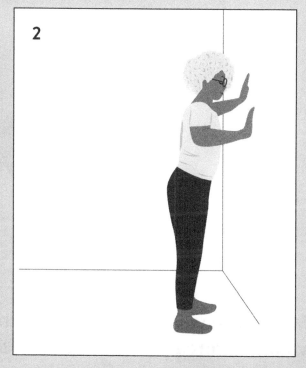

1. Begin by positioning your body as in the traditional wall pushup, with your hands staggered (right hand at shoulder height and the left hand above your shoulder). Ensure your legs are hip-distance apart.

2. Inhale and engage your core.

3. Exhale as you lower your chest to the wall, ensuring your body's alignment remains straight.

4. Inhale to push back up to the start and repeat.

WALL-ASSISTED PECTORAL STRETCH
Hold for 20 seconds on each side, 2 sets

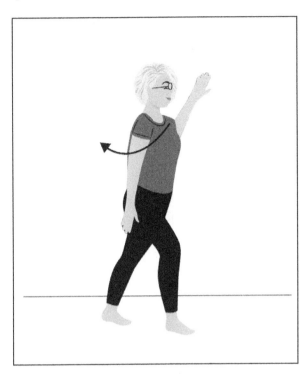

19

1. **Stand with your left side facing the wall. Bend your left arm and place your left forearm on the wall, at shoulder height.**

2. **Step forward with your right leg, and at the same time, slightly rotate your left shoulder forward and out towards the right. It's important that your forearm doesn't move and that all the stretching motion is coming from your left pectoral muscle /left side of your chest.**

3. **Hold for 20 seconds, then relax. Repeat one more time on the same side.**

4. **Turn around, switch sides and do the pectoral stretch twice on that side too.**

Our chest muscles are prone to becoming tight due to sitting for a long time and hunching over. By using the wall to stretch your chest muscles, you'll be able to loosen the muscles, decrease any pain caused by the tightness, and increase your flexibility and mobility in your upper body.

WALL SHOULDER EXTENSION STRETCH
Hold for 20 seconds, 2 sets

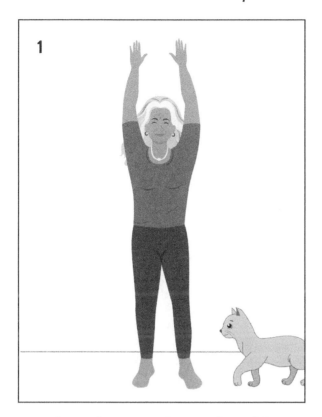

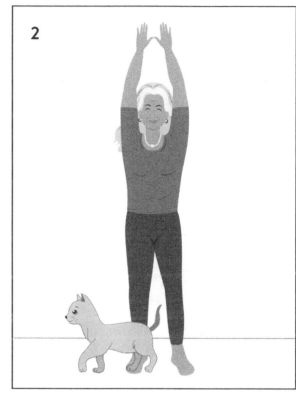

1. Stand with your feet shoulder-width apart and your back against the wall.

2. Extend your arms above your head with the backs of your hands resting against the wall.

3. Keeping your elbows straight, slide your hands up the wall until you feel a stretch in your shoulders.

4. Hold for 20 seconds. Do 2 sets.

FINISH WITH 2 - 3 MINUTES OF DEEP LATERAL BREATHING Page 15

BEGIN WITH 1 MINUTE OF DEEP LATERAL BREATHING

Page
15

NECK ROLLS
5 times in each direction

20

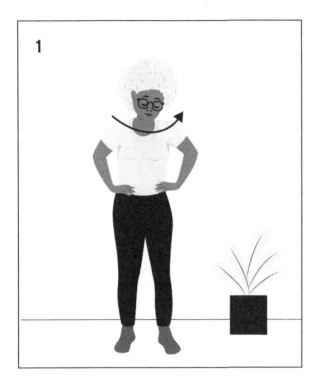

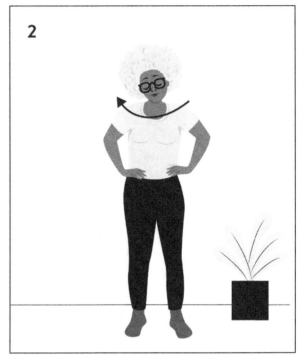

1. Stand tall with your hands on your waist and your head facing forward. Ensure your shoulders are away from your ears and your core supports your posture.

2. Tuck your chin down towards your neck and slowly roll your head to the left, until your chin is above your left shoulder, and you're looking slightly upwards and behind you.

3. Drop your chin, and tuck it in as you slowly roll your head down and to the right, until your chin is above your right shoulder, and you're looking slightly upwards and behind you on the right side.

4. Repeat in alternating directions 5 times.

SEATED ARM CIRCLES

10 times in each direction, 2 sets

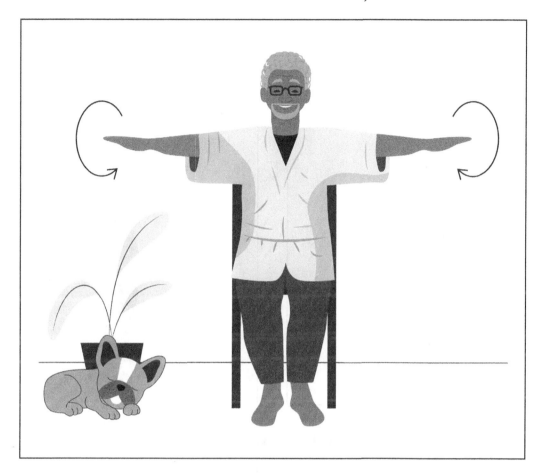

20

1. Sit in your chair with a lengthened spine. Ensure your core muscles are engaged.

2. Extend your arms to make a "T" shape with your palms facing the floor.

3. Start making small circles from your shoulder joint with your arms circling to the back. Continue doing this, making your circles larger each time for 30 seconds.

4. Lower your arms and shake them out.

5. Lift them back up to the "T" shape and repeat with your circles going to the front for 30 seconds.

6. Repeat 10 times in each direction and do 2 sets.

WALL SLIDES WITH HEAD NODS
15 to 20 times, 2 sets

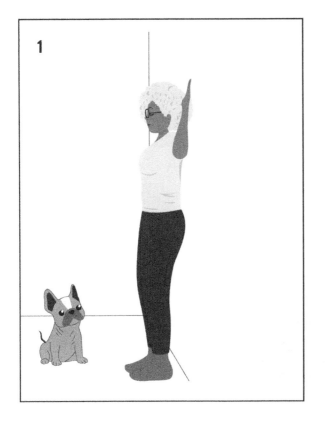 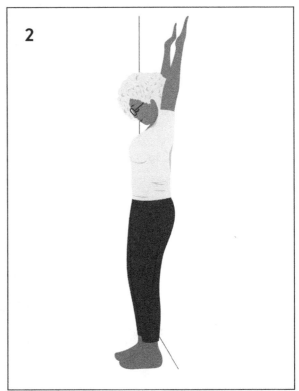

1. Stand with your back against the wall and feet shoulder-width apart.

2. Position your arms in the wall slide position with your elbows bent 90 degrees. Your forearms and the backs of your hands should be resting against your wall.

3. Slowly slide your arms up the wall as you nod. Tuck your chin into your chest.

4. Slide your arms back down, lift your head back to its starting position, and repeat 15 - 20 times. Do 2 sets.

WALL SIDE LEG LIFTS
10 to 15 times on each side

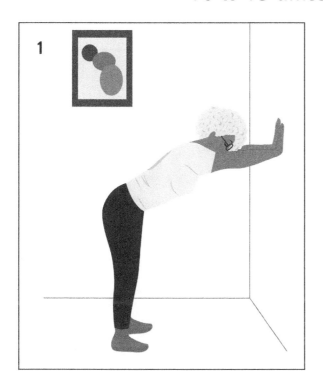 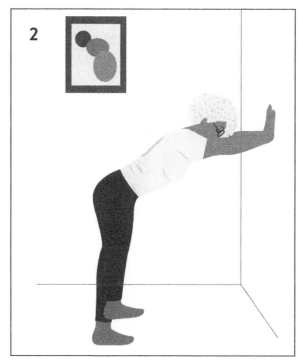

1. **Stand facing the wall.**

2. **Take a few steps back from the wall.**

3. **Bend forward to rest your hands on your wall for support. Your back should parallel the ceiling, and your toes should face the wall.**

4. **Engage your core and lift your leg to the side as high as it will go.**

5. **Lower it down halfway, then lift it back up.**

Leg lifts work your entire core muscles as you lift your legs to the side, including the ab muscles that make up our "six-pack" in the front, as well as our obliques, our back muscles, our diaphragm, our pelvic floor, our hip flexors and our glute (butt) muscles. In other words, these are great for us in all sorts of ways!

WALL-ASSISTED CROSS-BODY SHOULDER STRETCH

Holding for 20 seconds, 5 sets on each side

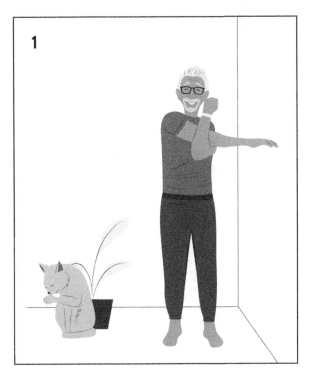
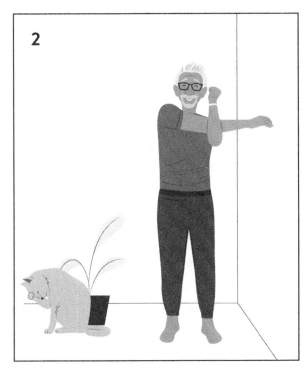

1. Stand about an arm's distance from your wall with your left side facing it.

2. Bring your right arm across your chest, keeping it straight, and place your hand against the wall for support.

3. Using your left hand, press against your right shoulder until you feel a stretch in your upper back and right shoulder.

4. Hold for 20 seconds, then switch to your left arm. Do it 5 sets.

WALL-ASSISTED INNER THIGH STRETCH
Holding for 20 seconds, 3 sets

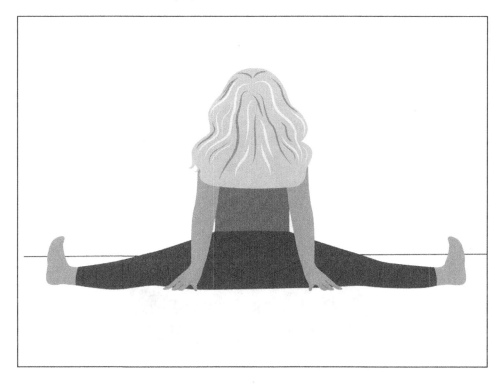

20

1. Sit facing your wall with your legs spread as wide as is comfortable.

2. Wiggle your bottom forward until the bottoms of your feet are against the wall. Engage your core to lengthen your spine.

3. Place your hands on your knees and gently press into them until you feel a stretch. Alternatively, you can place your hands on the floor and lean into them as you lower your upper body.

4. Hold for 20 seconds. Relax and repeat. Do 3 sets.

For the Wall-Assisted inner thigh stretch, you will want plenty of space to perform it—a corner may also work well.

NOTE: This is one of the few exercises that's on the floor. If you don't feel comfortable, then feel free to skip until you're ready.

FINISH WITH 2 - 3 MINUTES OF DEEP LATERAL BREATHING
Page
15

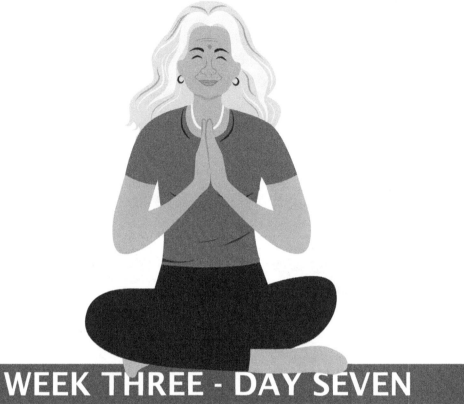

21

WEEK THREE - DAY SEVEN

REST DAY

WEEK FOUR - DAY ONE

BEGIN WITH 1 MINUTE OF DEEP LATERAL BREATHING Page 15

NECK ROLL AND STRETCH
5 times on each side

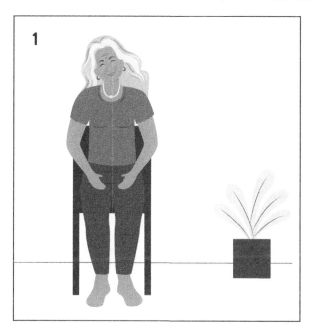

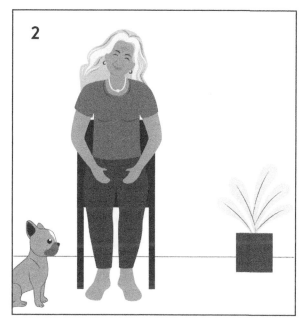

1. Sit in your chair with relaxed shoulders. Rest your hands on your lap.

2. Slowly tilt your head to the right to feel a stretch in the left side of your neck. Hold for a moment.

3. Gently roll your head forward while tucking in your chin to look down. Hold for a moment.

4. While keeping your chin tucked, turn your head to the right to look at your shoulder. Hold for a moment.

5. Turn your head back to the center to look back down at your lap, then bring your head back up to look forward.

6. Repeat on the left side.

7. Continue until you have completed this exercise five times on each side.

This exercise has a small rolling component, and will have you stretching the back of your neck as you roll it from right to left. It can be done standing or sitting in a chair. If you choose to stand, keep your legs about hip-width apart.

CALF RAISES
20 times

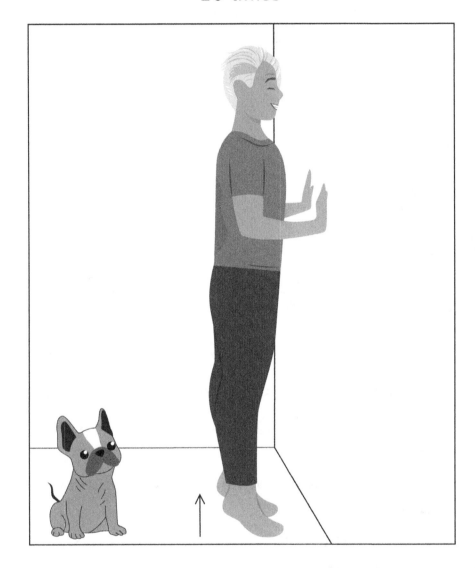

1. **Stand facing your wall with your feet about hip-width apart. Engage your core muscles to lengthen your spine. Your feet should be facing forward.**

2. **Lift your heels off the floor.**

3. **Lower and repeat up to 20 times.**

Strengthening your calves has plenty of benefits but, most importantly, having strong calves benefits your ankles and feet.

WALL SQUATS WITH HEEL RAISES
8 to 10 times, 2 sets

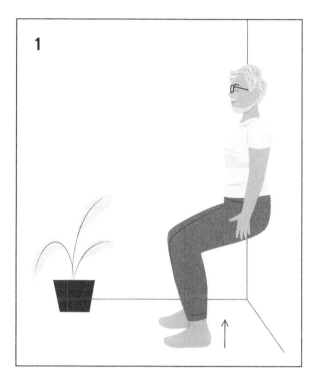 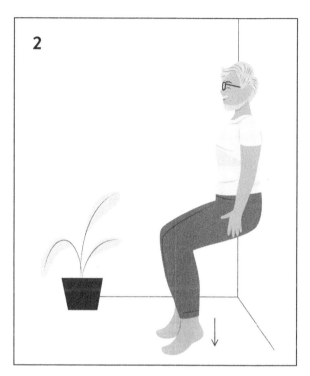

1. **Lean against the wall with your knees bent. Walk them out until you are "sitting" on an invisible chair.**

2. **Engage your core to ensure your back remains straight and flat against the wall.**

3. **Shift your weight to the balls of your feet to lift your heels.**

4. **Hold for three seconds, then lower, and stand back up.**

5. **Repeat steps three and four, 8 - 10 times. Do 2 sets.**

The wall squat combined with a heel raise targets all of the muscles a traditional squat does but with a twist. In this squat variation, raising your heels will further activate your quads as your knees will extend more over your toes in the squat position, aiding you to go just a little deeper.

WALL PUSH-UPS
5 - 10 times

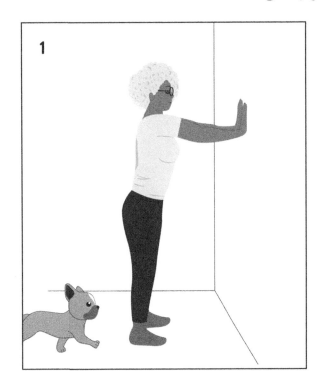

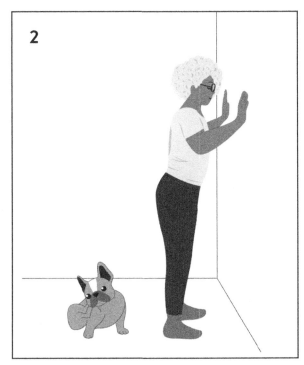

1. Stand no more than two feet from the wall, adjusting the distance according to your fitness level. You'll want to be closer to the wall if traditional push-ups are hard for you.

2. Place your hands on the wall at your shoulder height, just a bit wider than your shoulder width, and fingers are pointing up to the ceiling. Adjust your legs to be hip-width apart.

3. Engage your core and inhale.

4. Exhale to lower your chest toward the wall.

5. Inhale to push back up to the start and repeat.

6. Continue until you have completed 5 - 10 push-ups.

ADVANCED EXERCISE

WEEK FOUR - DAY ONE

INCLINE PUSH-UPS
5 - 10 times

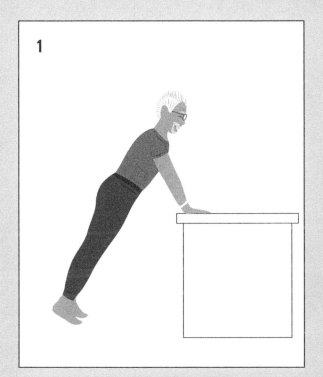
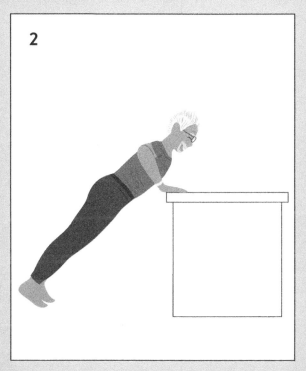

22

1. Begin by facing your flat surface with your hands on the edge, shoulder-width apart. Step back until your body makes a straight line from the top of your head to your heels. Ensure your arms are extended.

2. Inhale and engage your core.

3. Exhale as you lower your chest to the surface.

4. Inhale to push back up to the start and repeat.

Unlike the other pushup exercises where you have been using a wall, this one is better done facing a sturdy, high surface such as a railing or a countertop, as the setup is similar to doing a traditional pushup on the floor.

OVERHEAD WALL CHEST STRETCH
Hold for 20 seconds, 2 sets

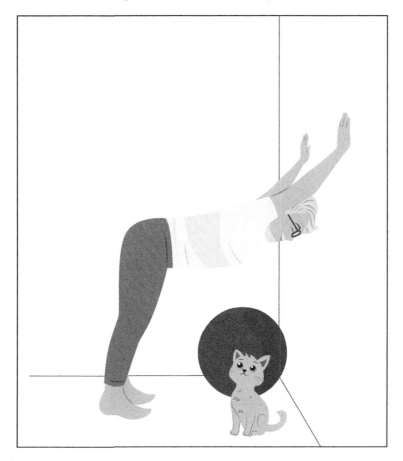

1. **Stand an arm's length away from your wall, facing it.**

2. **Raise your arms above your head. Place your hands against the wall.**

3. **Maintaining your straight arms, lean forward to press your chest against the wall, stopping when you feel a stretch in your upper chest.**

4. **Hold for 20 seconds, then relax and repeat. Do 2 sets.**

WEEK FOUR - DAY ONE

SEATED HIP FLEXOR STRETCH
Holding for 20 seconds, 2 sets

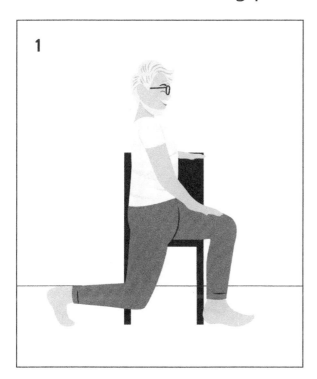

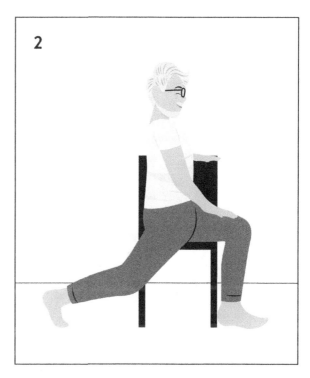

1. Sit sideways in your chair with your left side facing the backrest.

2. Extend your right leg as far behind you as possible until you feel a stretch in your hip and thigh. The ball of your foot should be placed flat on the floor, and your heel should be lifted. Ensure your spine is tall by engaging your core muscles.

3. Hold for 20 seconds.

4. Bring your leg back in, then switch sides. Do 2 sets.

FINISH WITH 2 - 3 MINUTES OF DEEP LATERAL BREATHING Page 15

LEG SWINGS
10 times with each leg

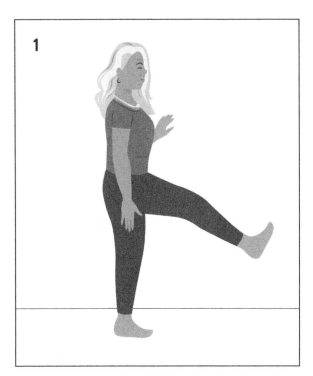

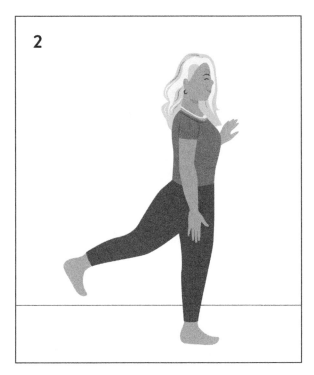

23

1. **Stand with your left side facing your wall. Engage your core muscles to keep you from losing your balance.**

2. **Keeping your left leg stationary, begin swinging your right leg forward and backward, aiming to swing higher each time.**

3. **Repeat 10 times in each direction, then switch sides.**

If you spend a significant amount of time sitting, it will impact your hip flexors because they become compressed. Over time, it can lead to pain and mobility issues. However, leg swings can help warm up and stretch the muscles and tendons in your hip joint, relieving any discomfort and removing your hips from a compressed position.

WEEK FOUR - DAY TWO

SEATED MARCHES
1 minute

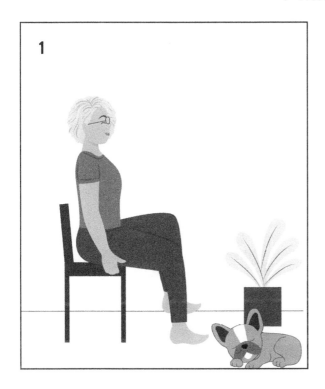 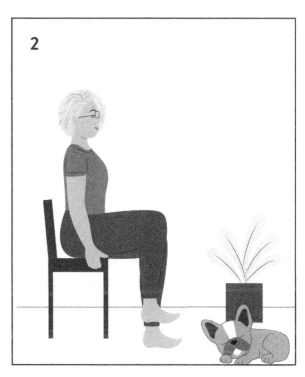

1. Sit in your chair near the front with your hands holding the sides of the seat for support.

2. Engage your core muscles to lengthen your spine.

3. Start lifting your left leg off the floor, then switch to your right in a marching movement.

4. Continue to march for a minute.

Seated marches will give you a quick boost of energy and cardio as they increase your heart rate. This exercise is great for a warm-up or any time during the day for movement.

SEATED SINGLE-LEG EXTENSION

10 reps on each side, 2 sets

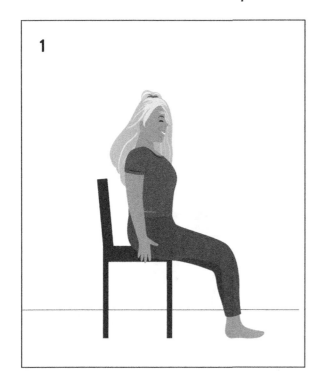
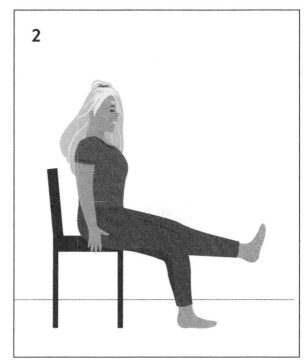

23

1. Sit near the edge of your seat with your legs hip-width apart.

2. Engage your core to lengthen your spine. Place your hands on either side of the chair seat. Take a deep breath in.

3. Exhale to lift your left leg. Stop when your leg is straight out from your hip. Lower and repeat 10 times.

4. Switch sides. Do 2 sets.

SINGLE-LEG WALL SQUAT
WITH (OR WITHOUT) STABILITY BALL

10 times, 2 sets

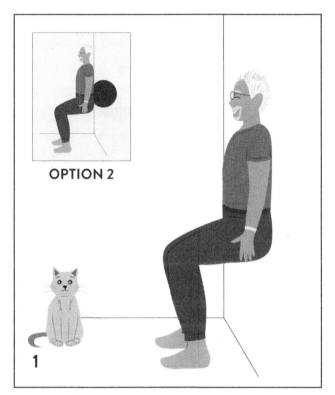

OPTION 2

1

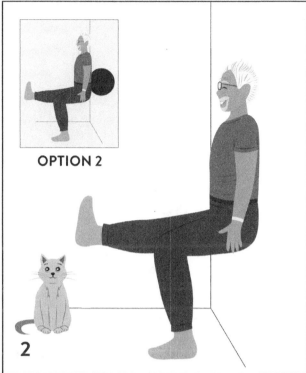

OPTION 2

2

23

1. Stand with your back against the wall.

2. Shift your weight to your left leg and then lift your right leg so that it's in front of you, with your foot flexed and pointing up to the ceiling.

3. Engage your core to lengthen your spine.

4. Press your back into the stability ball as you inhale.

5. Exhale and lower into the squat with your right leg.

6. Inhale to stand back up and repeat 10 times. Do 2 sets.

NOTE: If this is too hard, just lift your right foot so that it's simply off the floor.

WALL PUSH-UPS
5 - 10 times

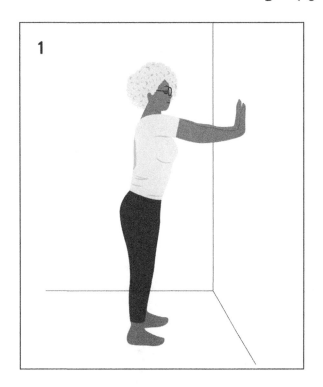 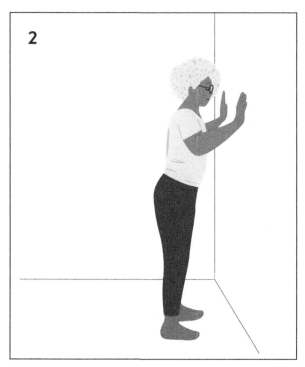

1. Stand no more than two feet from the wall, adjusting the distance according to your fitness level. You'll want to be closer to the wall if traditional push-ups are hard for you.

2. Place your hands on the wall at your shoulder height, just a bit wider than your shoulder width, and fingers are pointing up to the ceiling. Adjust your legs to be hip-width apart.

3. Engage your core and inhale.

4. Exhale to lower your chest toward the wall.

5. Inhale to push back up to the start and repeat.

6. Continue until you have completed 5 - 10 push-ups.

BONUS EXERCISE

WEEK FOUR - DAY TWO

ONE-ARM WALL PUSH-UPS

5 reps on both sides

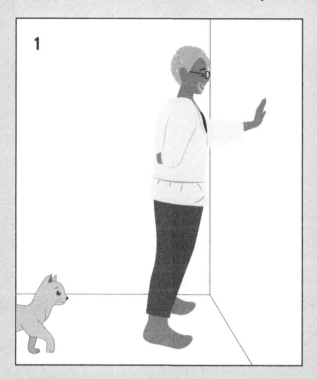
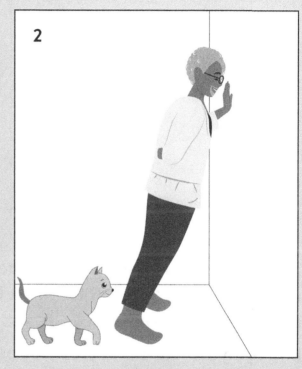

1. Begin by positioning your body as in the traditional wall push-up, with your left hand against the wall a little wider than your shoulders. Ensure your legs are hip-distance apart.

2. Place your right arm behind your back.

3. Inhale and engage your core.

4. Exhale as you lower your chest to the wall, keeping your elbow close to your body.

5. Inhale to push back up to the start, and repeat 10 times. Then switch to your right arm.

WALL ROLL-DOWNS
5 times

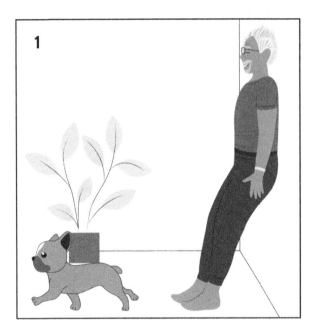 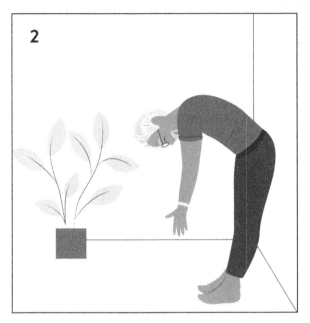

1. **Stand with your back against the wall, ensuring your butt touches it. Have your feet about 6 to 10 inches from the wall. Your arms should dangle beside you with your shoulders away from your ears.**

2. **Engage your core muscles as you inhale deeply.**

3. **Exhale and slowly nod your head as you slowly roll down as far as possible. Ensure your butt stays on the wall while your upper back moves away. Your arms should also hang as you roll down; allow them, along with your head, neck, and shoulders, to relax. You may also want to scoop your abs in further to engage them as you roll down.**

4. **When you reach your furthest point, take another inhale. Feel how your back is curved between your torso's upper, middle, and lower sections. You may also feel a stretch in your hamstrings.**

5. **Exhale and slowly roll back up, picturing your vertebrae stacking on top of one another. Engage your abs to assist you as you go. Repeat 5 times.**

OVERHEAD WALL CHEST STRETCH

Hold for 20 seconds, 2 sets

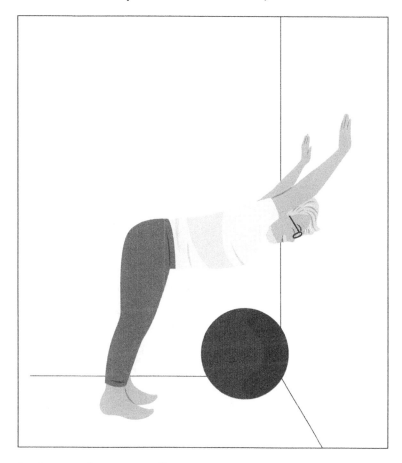

23

1. Stand an arm's length away from your wall, facing it.

2. Raise your arms above your head. Place your hands against the wall.

3. Maintaining your straight arms, lean forward to press your chest against the wall, stopping when you feel a stretch in your upper chest.

4. Hold for 20 seconds, then relax and repeat. Do 2 sets.

FINISH WITH 2 - 3 MINUTES OF DEEP LATERAL BREATHING Page **15**

ANKLE CIRCLES
5 times on each side

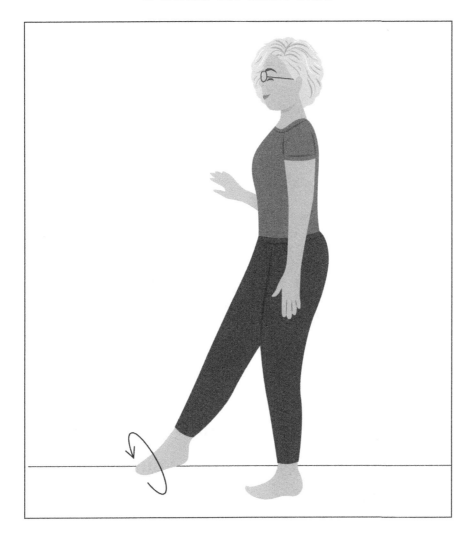

1. Stand tall next to your wall with your right hand resting against it for support.

2. Extend your right leg with your heel a few inches above the floor.

3. Make circles with your foot clockwise 10 times, then counterclockwise.

4. Switch legs.

5. Repeat 5 times in each direction.

CALF RAISES
20 times

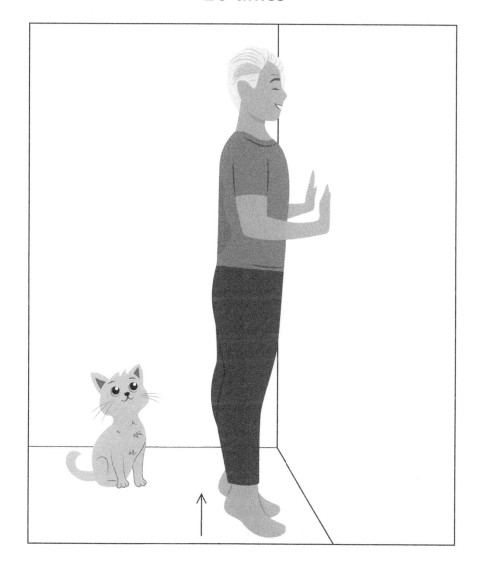

24

1. **Stand facing your wall with your feet about hip-width apart. Engage your core muscles to lengthen your spine. Your feet should be facing forward.**

2. **Lift your heels off the floor.**

3. **Lower and repeat up to 20 times.**

Strengthening your calves has plenty of benefits but, most importantly, having strong calves benefits your ankles and feet.

TRADITIONAL WALL PLANK
Hold for 10 - 30 seconds

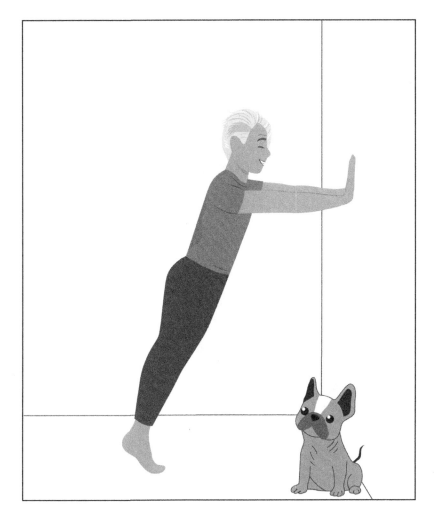

24

1. **Start with your hands resting against the wall, your arms straight, and your legs hip-width apart and slightly back from the wall to put your body in a straight diagonal.**
   To make this exercise more challenging, then instead of having your arms straight, bend them and rest your forearms against the wall.

2. **Engage your core and try to hold for as long as possible, but aim for at least 10 seconds and work up from there.**

Planks have plenty of benefits, especially for strengthening your core muscles. Using the wall will provide you with more stabilization for your core while helping you find a better balance.

SIDE PLANK WITH ROTATION

2 -3 times on each side

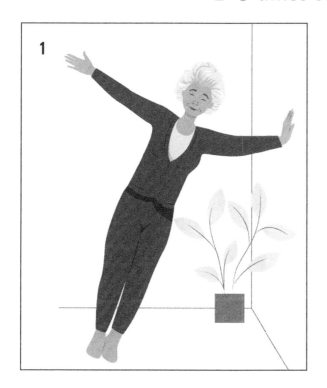 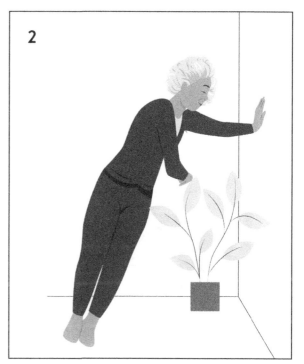

1. Start in the side plank position against the wall, leaning against your left arm.

2. Extend your right arm beside you to make half of a "T" shape.

3. Move your right arm down and under your upper body as if you're going to hug your belly.

4. Untwist to return to the starting position, extend your arm beside you, then repeat 10 times on each side.

WEEK FOUR - DAY THREE

SEATED SCISSOR LEGS
15 times

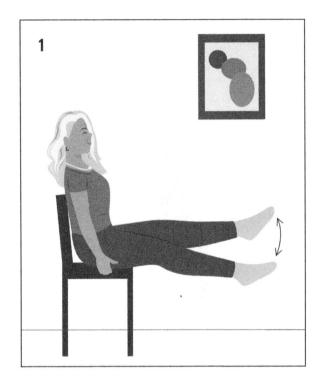 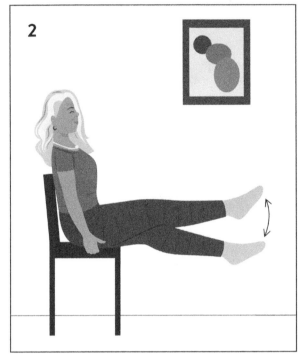

1. Sit in your chair with your bottom slightly forward from the middle. Support yourself by placing your hands on either side of your chair seat.

2. Lift your legs straight in front of you, keeping your ankles slightly relaxed.

3. Engage your core muscles to lengthen your spine.

4. Cross your right leg over the left, then switch, continuing to alternate between legs. Ensure that as you scissor your legs, your shoulders are not creeping up to your ears.

5. Continue the exercise for up to one minute.

WEEK FOUR - DAY THREE

WALL-ASSISTED SIDE BEND

Hold for 20 seconds on each side

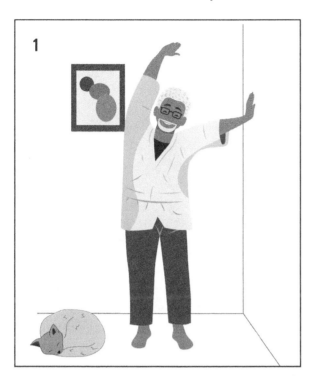 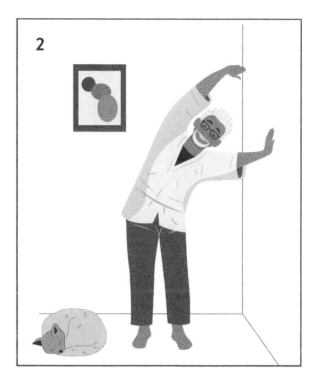

1. Stand with your left side facing the wall and your legs hip-distance apart.

2. Raise your left arm to shoulder height and rest your left hand against the wall.

3. Raise your right arm over your head, and stretch it as far as you can towards the wall.

4. Hold for 20 seconds. You should feel the stretch along the length of your right side, as well as a crunch in your left side abdomen muscles.

5. Switch sides and do the same stretch, holding for 20 seconds.

WEEK FOUR - DAY THREE

WALL-ASSISTED CALF STRETCH
Hold for 20 seconds on each side

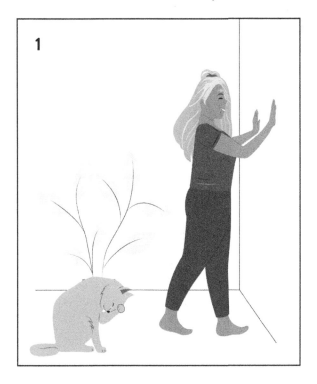

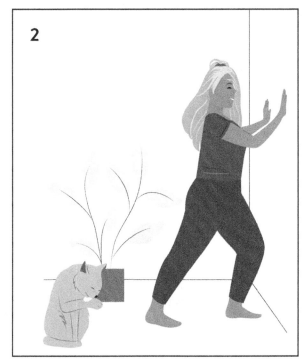

1. Stand an arm's length away from the wall, facing it.

2. Rest your hands against the wall at shoulder height.

3. Step your right foot back and bend your left leg. Ensure your right heel stays on the ground. If you can't get your heel onto the floor, shorten the distance.

4. Hold the stretch for 20 seconds, then switch legs.

FINISH WITH 2 - 3 MINUTES OF DEEP LATERAL BREATHING Page 15

BEGIN WITH 1 MINUTE OF DEEP LATERAL BREATHING
Page
15

NECK ROLL AND STRETCH
5 times on each side

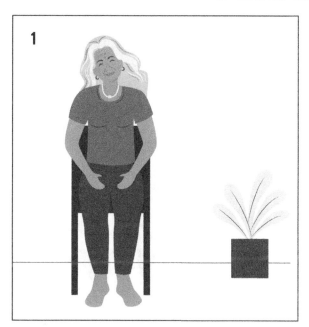
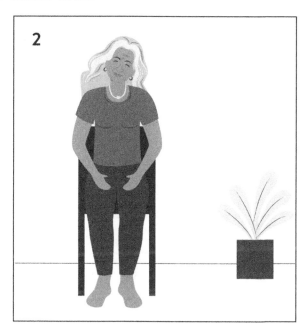

25

1. Sit in your chair with relaxed shoulders. Rest your hands on your lap.

2. Slowly tilt your head to the right to feel a stretch in the left side of your neck. Hold for a moment.

3. Gently roll your head forward while tucking in your chin to look down. Hold for a moment.

4. While keeping your chin tucked, turn your head to the right to look at your shoulder. Hold for a moment.

5. Turn your head back to the center to look back down at your lap, then bring your head back up to look forward.

6. Repeat on the left side.

7. Continue until you have completed this exercise five times on each side.

This exercise has a small rolling component, and will have you stretching the back of your neck as you roll it from right to left. It can be done standing or sitting in a chair. If you choose to stand, keep your legs about hip-width apart.

WRIST CIRCLES

30 seconds - 1 minute in each direction, 2 sets

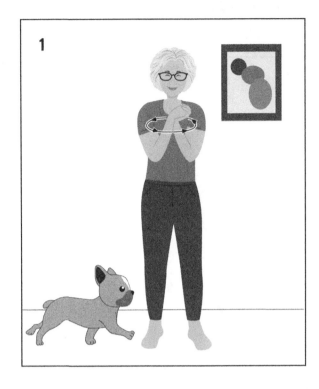 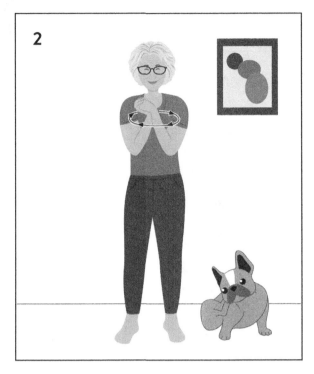

1. Clasp your hands together, interlocking your fingers.

2. Rotate your wrists clockwise for 30 seconds to 1 minute. Then, switch directions. Do 2 sets.

Our wrists are used more often than we realize every day. By performing wrist circles, you can help maintain your wrists' flexibility and range of motion.

WALL SLIDES WITH HEAD NODS
15 to 20 times, 2 sets

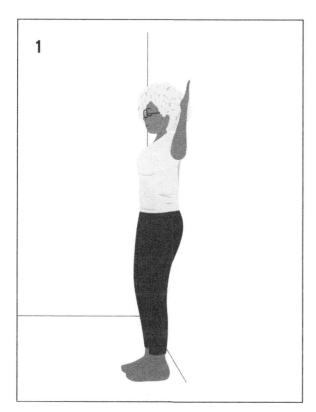 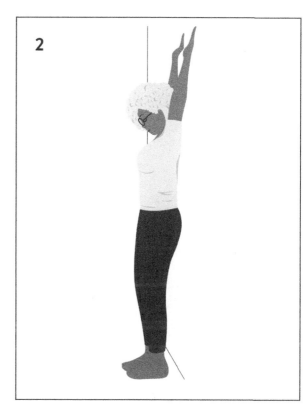

1. Stand with your back against the wall and feet shoulder-width apart.

2. Position your arms in the wall slide position with your elbows bent 90 degrees. Your forearms and the backs of your hands should be resting against your wall.

3. Slowly slide your arms up the wall as you nod. Tuck your chin into your chest.

4. Slide your arms back down, lift your head back to its starting position, and repeat 15 - 20 times. Do 2 sets.

WALL PUSH-UPS
5 - 10 times

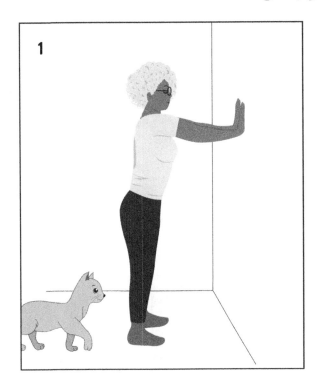 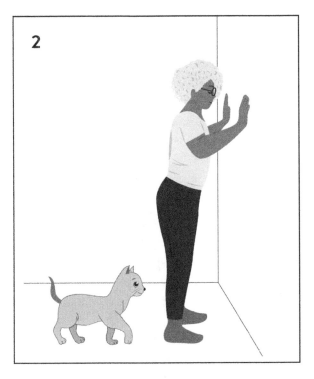

1. Stand no more than two feet from the wall, adjusting the distance according to your fitness level. You'll want to be closer to the wall if traditional push-ups are hard for you.

2. Place your hands on the wall at your shoulder height, just a bit wider than your shoulder width, and fingers are pointing up to the ceiling. Adjust your legs to be hip-width apart.

3. Engage your core and inhale.

4. Exhale to lower your chest toward the wall.

5. Inhale to push back up to the start and repeat.

6. Continue until you have completed 5 - 10 push-ups.

BONUS EXERCISE

WEEK FOUR - DAY FOUR

WIDE-GRIP WALL PUSH-UPS

3 - 5 reps

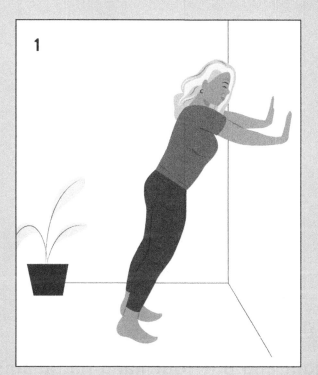
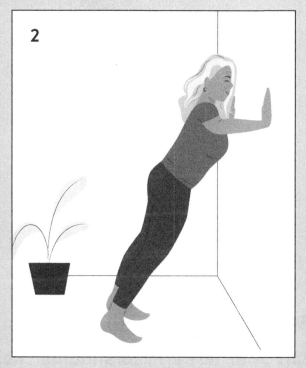

1. Begin by positioning your body as in the traditional wall push-up, but now place your hands wider than your shoulders (about 6 inches past each of your shoulders). Ensure your legs are hip-distance apart.

2. Inhale and engage your core.

3. Exhale as you lower your chest to the wall, bending your elbows to the sides of your body.

4. Inhale to push back up to the start and repeat 3 - 5 times.

WALL CHEST STRETCH
Hold for 20 seconds on each side

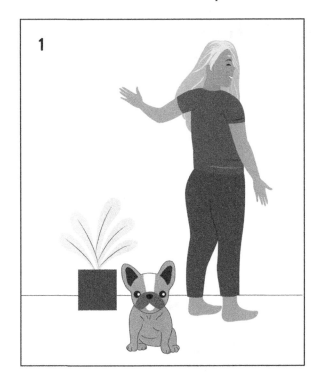 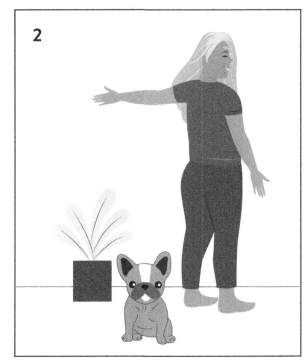

1. Stand an arm's length away from the wall.

2. Lift your left arm to shoulder height and put your hand flat against the wall, but slightly behind you and at a 90 degree angle.

3. Slowly turn your body away from the wall (to the right), keeping your hand on the wall, until you feel a stretch in your shoulder and chest. (Remember not to go further than your body is able!)

4. Hold for 20 seconds, then switch to your right side.

Our chest muscles are prone to becoming tight due to sitting for a long time and hunching over. By using the wall to stretch your chest muscles, you'll be able to loosen the muscles, decrease any pain caused by the tightness, and increase your flexibility and mobility in your upper body.

WALL-ASSISTED COBRA STRETCH
Holding for 20 seconds, 3 - 5 sets

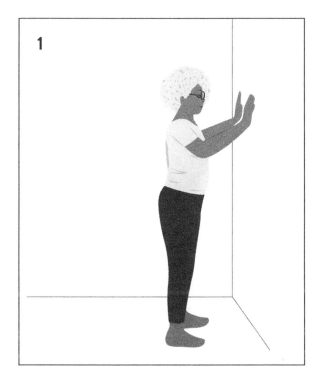

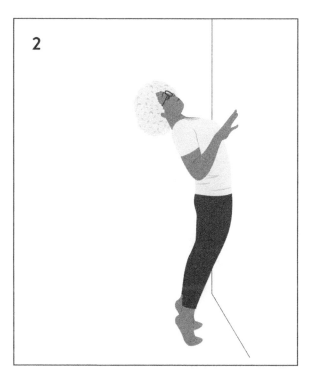

25

1. Stand an arm's length away from your wall, facing it.

2. Raise your hands to your shoulder height and rest them against the wall.

3. Press your hips forward to arch your back, lifting your chest to the ceiling. Tilt your gaze upwards.

4. Hold for 20 seconds, then relax and repeat three to five more times.

FINISH WITH 2 - 3 MINUTES OF DEEP LATERAL BREATHING Page 15

BEGIN WITH 1 MINUTE OF DEEP LATERAL BREATHING Page **15**

MARCHING
1 minute

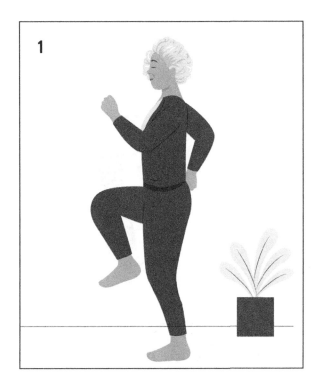

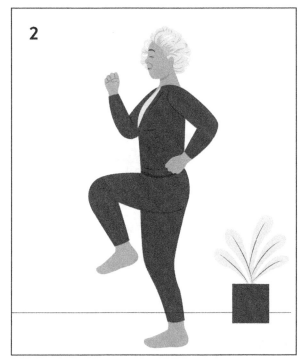

1. **Stand on your yoga mat with your feet hip-width apart. Engage your core muscles to straighten your spine. Your feet should be facing the front.**

2. **Lift your right leg as high as possible while simultaneously lifting your left arm with a bent elbow. Lower your leg and arm and repeat on the other side with your opposite arm and leg.**

3. **Continue alternating your legs until you've completed 12 to 15 on each side, or do up to 1 minute.**

Get a boost of cardio with this warm-up exercise! Marching will help to boost your heart rate and increase the mobility and flexibility in your hips and quadriceps.

TORSO TWISTS
1 minute

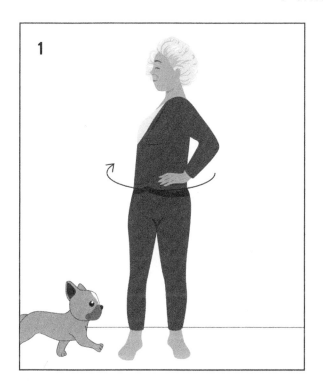
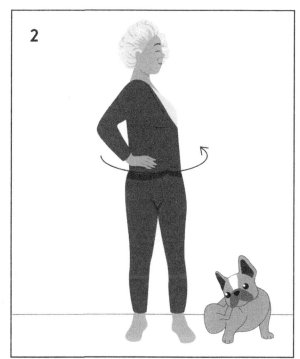

1. Stand tall with your feet hip-width apart and your hands on your waist.

2. Keeping your feet planted, twist your torso to the right as far as you can go, then twist the other way. Engage your core muscles and keep your feet planted on the floor so that the stretch is focused on your torso.

3. Repeat 5 to 10 times in each direction, or do more for up to a full minute.

TRADITIONAL WALL PLANK
Hold for 10 - 30 seconds

26

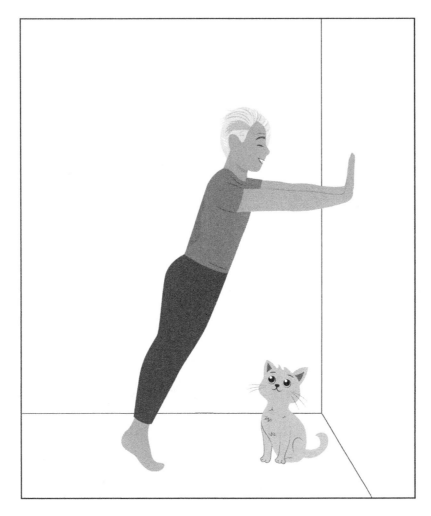

1. **Start with your hands resting against the wall, your arms straight, and your legs hip-width apart and slightly back from the wall to put your body in a straight diagonal.**
To make this exercise more challenging, then instead of having your arms straight, bend them and rest your forearms against the wall.

2. **Engage your core and try to hold for as long as possible, but aim for at least 10 seconds and work up from there.**

Planks have plenty of benefits, especially for strengthening your core muscles. Using the wall will provide you with more stabilization for your core while helping you find a better balance.

BONUS EXERCISE

WEEK FOUR - DAY FIVE

WALL PLANK WITH KNEE TUCK
5 - 10 reps on each side

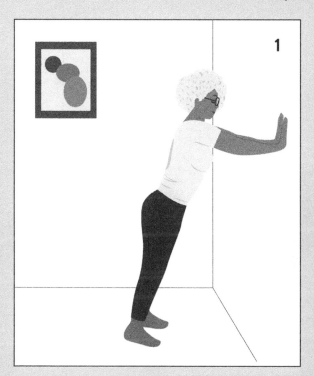
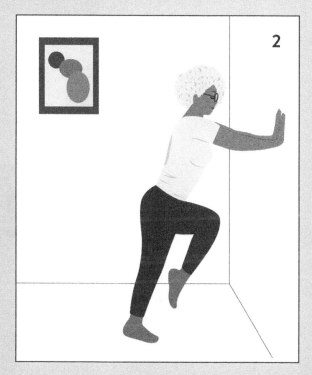

26

1. Start with your hands resting against the wall, your arms straight, and your legs hip-width apart and slightly back from the wall to put your body in a straight diagonal.

2. Engage your core muscles and ensure your shoulders are not rising to your ears.

3. Bend your left leg and bring your knee up towards your chest, so that your foot is off the floor, with your toes pointing downwards. Hold the position for a second, then lower your foot back to the ground and switch legs.

4. Continue alternating between legs, 5 - 10 times.

SEATED LEG CIRCLES

10 reps on each side, 2 sets

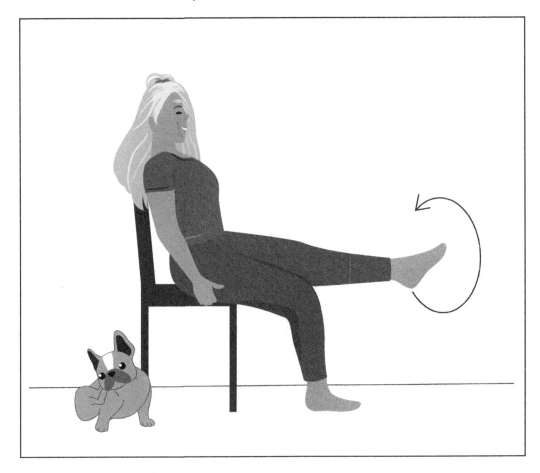

1. Sit forward in your chair, with your hands on the sides of the seat.

2. Lean into the back of the chair until your shoulders rest against your backrest. Keep your core engaged.

3. Extend your left leg to your hip's level.

4. Leading with your toes, slowly draw a large circle, then do it again going counterclockwise. Switch legs.

5. Continue alternating directions, both legs 10 times. Do 2 sets.

OVERHEAD WALL CHEST STRETCH
Hold for 20 seconds, 2 sets

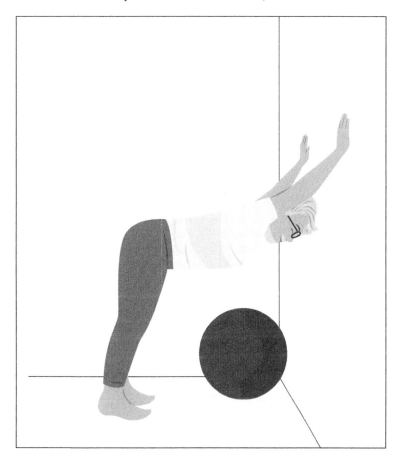

26

1. Stand an arm's length away from your wall, facing it.

2. Raise your arms above your head. Place your hands against the wall.

3. Maintaining your straight arms, lean forward to press your chest against the wall, stopping when you feel a stretch in your upper chest.

4. Hold for 20 seconds, then relax and repeat. Do 2 sets.

WALL-ASSISTED COBRA STRETCH
Holding for 20 seconds, 3 - 5 sets

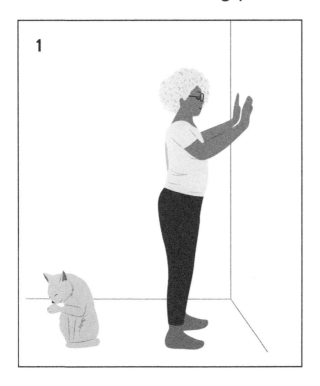

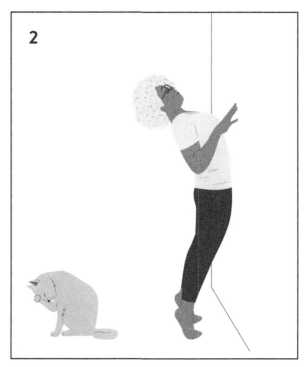

1. Stand an arm's length away from your wall, facing it.

2. Raise your hands to your shoulder height and rest them against the wall.

3. Press your hips forward to arch your back, lifting your chest to the ceiling. Tilt your gaze upwards.

4. Hold for 20 seconds, then relax and repeat three to five more times.

FINISH WITH 2 - 3 MINUTES OF DEEP LATERAL BREATHING Page 15

BEGIN WITH 1 MINUTE OF DEEP LATERAL BREATHING Page
15

ARM SWINGS
10 times in each direction

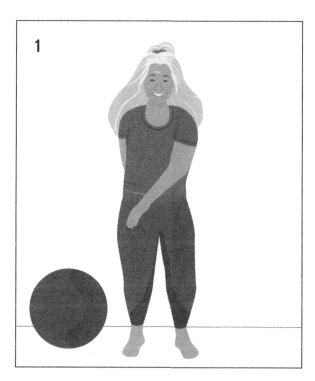

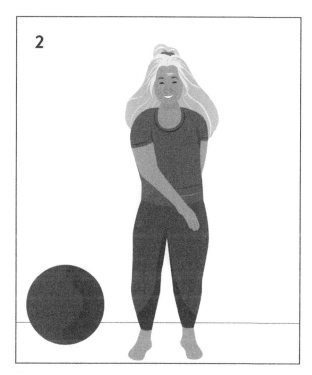

1. Stand with a tall spine and your feet wider than your shoulders. Allow your hands to hang loosely by your side.

2. Turn your torso to the right allowing your arms to swing across and around your body.

3. Turn in the other direction, repeating 10 times each way.

WALL PELVIC TILT
10 times, 2 sets

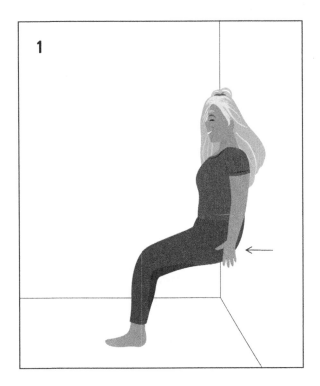 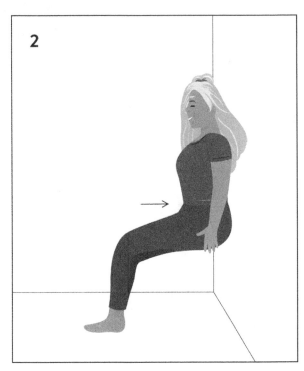

27

1. **Stand facing away from the wall and lean your back to rest against it. Ensure your knees have a slight bend to them.**

2. **Take a deep inhale.**

3. **On the exhale, tilt your pelvis up and away from the wall, straightening the natural curve of your lower back. You may find your lower back touches the wall, which is good. That's the goal of the tilt.**

4. **Tilt your pelvis to return to the starting position on your next inhale.**

5. **Repeat 10 times and do 2 sets.**

A pelvic tilt exercise can help address issues with your posture which can decrease back pain and strengthen your core.

WALL SLIDES WITH EXTERNAL ROTATION
15 to 20 times, 2 sets

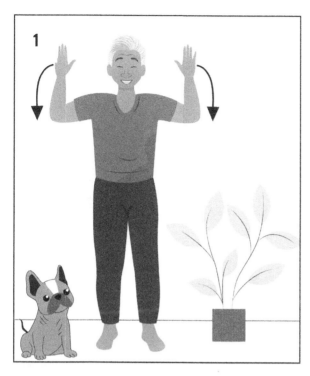

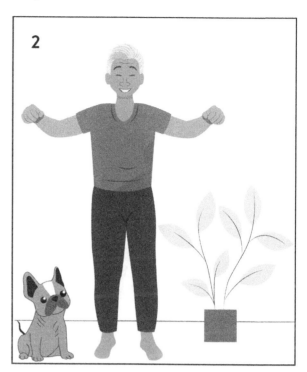

27

1. Stand with your back facing the wall, and with your feet about a foot away from the wall.

2. Put your hips and shoulders up against the wall, making sure that you don't arch your back too far away from the wall, and tuck your stomach in. Keep your elbows and forearms against the wall.

3. In a controlled manner, slowly rotate your forearms forward in a downward motion towards the floor. Keep your wrists in line with your forearms.

4. Stop when your forearms are at a 90 degree angle (basically at your natural shoulder / upper chest height). Then rotate your forearms back up, keeping your wrists inline, until your forearms are up against the wall again. Repeat. Do 2 sets of 15 - 20 times.

You should feel this in exercise in the back of your shoulders, and right at the join of your arm to your armpit. It's a fantastic exercise to increase the flexibility in your shoulders, which will give you better posture with your shoulders held back!

STANDING WALL CRUNCHES
10 times, 1 or 2 sets

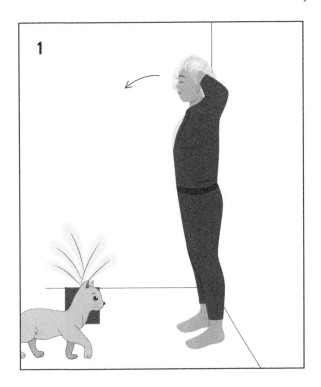 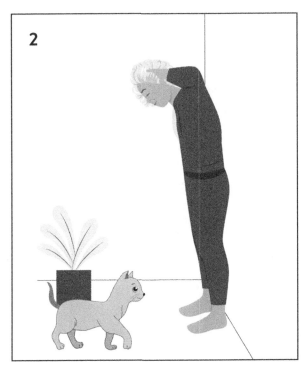

27

1. Stand about six to eight inches from your wall with your legs hip-width apart. Rest your hips, mid and upper back, and your head against the wall, ensuring your lower back and neck are not touching it. Place your hands against the back of your head.

2. Engage your abs and fold forward, starting with your upper back. Continue to bend at your waist as you push your ribs back to have your lower back touch the wall. Ensure you are breathing out as you contract your abs.

3. Inhale to return to the starting position. Repeat the crunch until you have completed between 10 and 20 reps.

Traditional crunches help build muscles in your abdominal region to improve your core's stability and protect your back from injury—but they can cause discomfort in your back or neck when performing them, which is why standing crunches are ideal.

SIDE PLANK WITH ROTATION
2 -3 times on each side

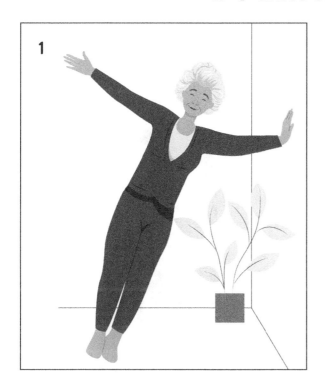 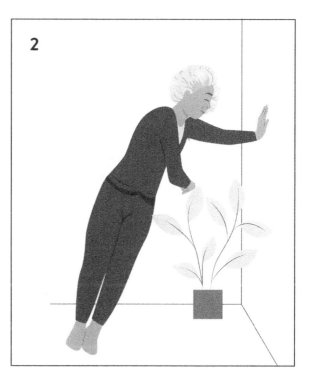

27

1. Start in the side plank position against the wall, leaning against your left arm.

2. Extend your right arm beside you to make half of a "T" shape.

3. Move your right arm down and under your upper body as if you're going to hug your belly.

4. Untwist to return to the starting position, extend your arm beside you, then repeat 10 times on each side.

SEATED MERMAID
10 times on each side

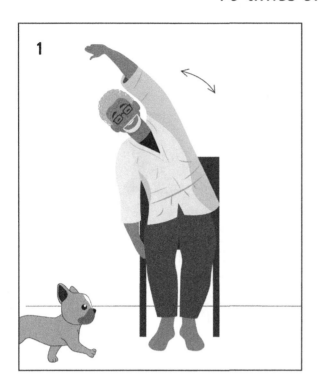 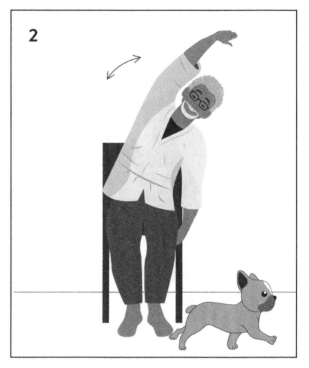

1. Sit in your chair with your legs about hip-width apart. Ensure your shoulders are back and down.

2. Place your right hand on the side of your chair as you reach your left arm overhead. Stretch to the right side until your left side feels a gentle stretch.

3. Hold the stretch and breathe into your ribcage. Return to the starting position on your last inhale and repeat on the right side.

4. Continue until you have completed 10 reps on each side.

WALL-ASSISTED PECTORAL STRETCH
Hold for 20 seconds on each side, 2 sets

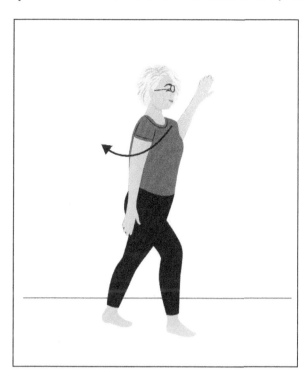

27

1. **Stand with your left side facing the wall. Bend your left arm and place your left forearm on the wall, at shoulder height.**

2. **Step forward with your right leg, and at the same time, slightly rotate your left shoulder forward and out towards the right. It's important that your forearm doesn't move and that all the stretching motion is coming from your left pectoral muscle /left side of your chest.**

3. **Hold for 20 seconds, then relax. Repeat one more time on the same side.**

4. **Turn around, switch sides and do the pectoral stretch twice on that side too.**

Our chest muscles are prone to becoming tight due to sitting for a long time and hunching over. By using the wall to stretch your chest muscles, you'll be able to loosen the muscles, decrease any pain caused by the tightness, and increase your flexibility and mobility in your upper body.

OVERHEAD WALL CHEST STRETCH
Hold for 20 seconds, 2 sets

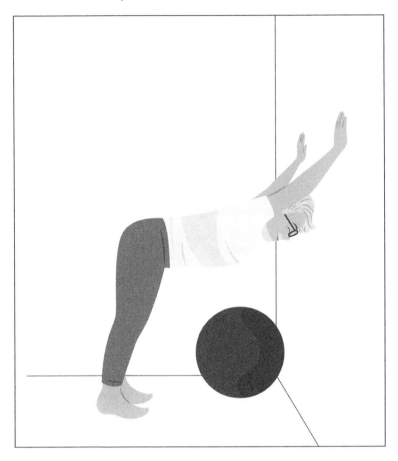

1. Stand an arm's length away from your wall, facing it.

2. Raise your arms above your head. Place your hands against the wall.

3. Maintaining your straight arms, lean forward to press your chest against the wall, stopping when you feel a stretch in your upper chest.

4. Hold for 20 seconds, then relax and repeat. Do 2 sets.

FINISH WITH 2 - 3 MINUTES OF DEEP LATERAL BREATHING Page 15

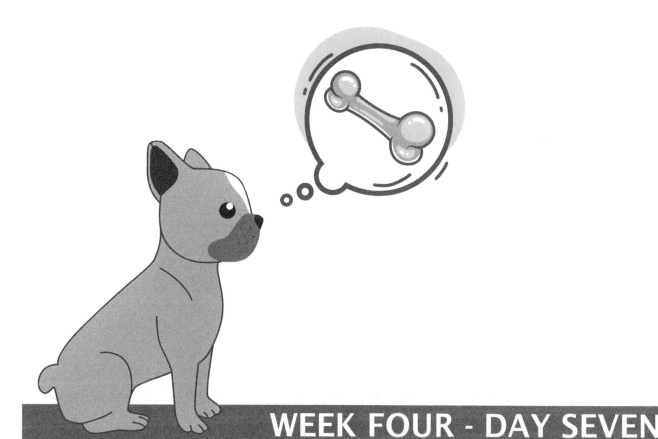

28

WEEK FOUR - DAY SEVEN

REST DAY

Congratulations! You've finished the first 28-Day loop! Now move on to your second round and start the 28-Day loop again.

This time, add in the Bonus exercises for an elevated challenge, and also more repetitions of the exercises for a longer duration in your exercise routine!

Do what you can, but keep building on your routine as you get more proficient.

And while you're building your exercise routine, read through the following chapters to incorporate nutrition and overall wellness activities to continue on your path to a vibrant lifestyle!

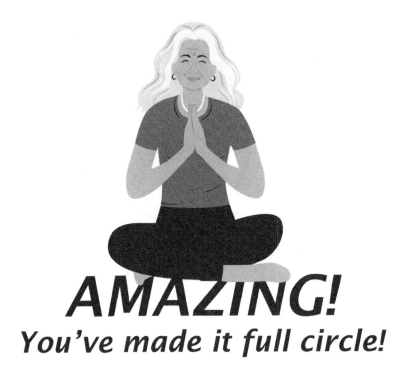

AMAZING!
You've made it full circle!

If this journey has been valuable to you, please make it possible for another to find it as well by leaving a ★★★★★ review!

Words are powerful, and your review could help change another person's fitness with that first small step, by getting this book into their hands. Thank you for your kindness, and now grab your meal planner and your wellness journal, as you round out your own fitness journey across the next few short chapters!

US CUSTOMERS, SCAN QR CODE:

GLOBAL CUSTOMERS, FOLLOW THESE STEPS:

1. Go to your Amazon "Your Orders" page ("Digital Orders" if you purchased the e-book)

2. Select "Wall Pilates for Seniors" by Ivy Thomas

3. Click on "WRITE A PRODUCT REVIEW" and describe your experience of this book.

AND THANK YOU!

CHAPTER 5:

BE THE FORCE YOU ARE, AND ADD OVERALL WELL-BEING TO YOUR EXERCISE!

It's exciting to feel fit and ready to take on the world! To increase that feeling, you need to look beyond exercise and add in eating well, and participating in healthful activities that will both stimulate your mind and relax your person.

Grab your meal planner and let's start with a basic look at food!

Nutritional and Dietary Activities

Eating well is a huge component to our overall health and our ability to move. What does eating well mean to you? Eating well, by definition, means you are eating a well-balanced diet to keep yourself healthy. Eating well helps you to reach or maintain a healthy weight, decreases your chances of developing a serious health condition such as heart disease and diabetes, and gives you the fuel you need to keep you energized in your workouts and throughout the day.

Maintaining a healthy diet seems to be so much more complex these days, but it doesn't need to be. Of course, nutritional needs differ from person to person, but these strategies will help you maintain a healthy diet and a healthy weight.

To start, focus on ensuring you eat nutrient-rich foods. These foods have higher vitamins and minerals, protein, carbohydrates, and fats you need to get the most of your calories.

These foods include:

- fruits and vegetables
- lentils and beans
- whole grains
- nuts and seeds
- low-fat dairy products
- lean protein, such as chicken and turkey

Unless your doctor tells you to avoid them altogether, eating well does not mean you need to cut out all of the "bad foods" like deep-fried foods and desserts—but you should limit them as they don't provide any nutritional value. You can also modify your cooking habits to be healthier and make French fries (or any other food) in an air fryer instead of in hot oil, and make desserts with stevia instead of with sugar.

In addition to eating nutrient-dense foods, ensuring you have enough fiber will also help you maintain a healthy digestive system and weight. More and more research has been coming out in the last decade about how integral our gut is to our overall health. When it's not working well, it can lead to many issues including constipation, weight gain, fatigue, etc.

As for how your gut health and fiber connect, think of fiber like a long sweeping broom taking out the things our body doesn't need. So, fruits and veggies are your best friend for giving you plenty of fiber. However, you can also get more fiber into your diet by eating:

- whole grains
- beans and lentils
- nuts and seeds
- oats and oat bran
- fiber supplements

Taking these factors into account for your nutrition side of your health, think about what your goals are. If your goal is to lose weight, eating well and making conscious decisions about what you are eating will help you with this. Ultimately, it all circles back to your gut health so when you take care of that, you'll be moving better, feel more energetic, and ready to take on the world.

Tips for Eating Well

So how do you ensure you keep eating well to maintain a healthy body? These tips should help:

- **Stick to a routine eating schedule:** Just like scheduling when you will be doing Wall Pilates, sticking to a regular eating schedule will be a good way to ensure you don't skip a meal accidentally.

- **Take a nutrition-focused cooking class:** Besides being therapeutic and social, a cooking class is one way to try out some new healthy recipes. This is also a great way to sharpen your mind as you learn a new skill, especially if the class has a cuisine you might not otherwise have ventured into making!

- **Eat with friends or family:** When possible, try to eat with friends and family. Eating with others can make eating more enjoyable and when you're talking and visiting at the table, it makes you eat more slowly and likely, less. Plus, if you happen to have a new recipe you've been wanting to try, this is a great time to share it with someone else!

Staying Hydrated

Eating nutrient-rich foods on a daily basis is not the only thing your body needs—you also must drink plenty of water. Water is vital to our bodily functions, such as lubricating our joints so they can move with ease and helping blood move to and through our hearts. By keeping our bodily systems moving, water not only hydrates us and keeps us running, but it can also help with weight loss goals.

If you want to get more water in your day, the good news is that there are some foods that have higher water content. So, while you're adding more nutrient-dense foods into your diet, you might want to include some of these foods into your meals and snacks as they are water-rich:

- strawberries
- cucumbers
- watermelon
- lettuce
- celery
- tomatoes
- soups
- broths
- stews

You can also add flavor to your water, such as lime, lemon, apple, cucumber, or berries.

The most important takeaway about staying hydrated is building it into your routine. Keep water with you all of the time, but also make it a habit to drink a glass of water when you wake up before you have tea or coffee. You should also try and have one glass before and with every meal.

Taking care of your nutrition and water intake will make you feel great, increase your energy and will work alongside your fitness routine to help you reach your healthiest weight!

Now that we've touched on nutrition, let's look at the other pillars of whole health: brain health, emotional / social health and spiritual or holistic wellness.

Mental and Cognitive Activities

Taking care of our brain health is another critical thing to do as we age, as so many factors can inhibit its ability to function. We can keep our minds sharp through various mental and cognitive activities, such as:

- **Playing brain-stimulating games:** the popular New York Times game, Wordle, is a good one for making your brain work as you try to decipher what the daily five-letter word is. Sudoku is another excellent brain game, as are chess, checkers, and memory games. Play a board game with your friends or family, including mahjong, Scrabble, Exit games (these are seriously fun, 'think outside the box' games), Rummoli - anything you like that's fun and is challenging to the way you think.

- **Learning new skills:** Our brains are always changing and evolving. When you learn new skills, you are making new connections and pathways in your brain. There are plenty of ways to learn, whether it's reading a book on a topic you don't know about, learning a new instrument, a new language, woodworking, stained glass, painting, etc. Whatever you have wanted to learn in the past, start learning it now and know that it's lighting up pathways in your brain and keeping you sharp!

- **Gardening activities:** Gardening is a pleasant leisure activity to do as it involves mental consistency alongside physical effort. You can do this on your own or with someone if you have difficulty lifting things or moving around.

- **Do a jigsaw puzzle:** Jigsaw puzzles are a mindful activity and one that doesn't take a lot of energy to do. This is something you can do with music or the TV on in the background as you work out putting the pieces together. I've even done chair exercises while doing puzzles - food for thought!

Emotional and Social Activities

Living alone isn't an ideal lifestyle for an older person's mental and physical well-being. I'm not trying to scare you, but living in a more isolated manner, in a Senior age bracket can lead to several concerning health risks, including:

- heart disease
- obesity
- depression
- cognitive decline
- Alzheimer's disease
- depression
- high blood pressure

Being social is good for mental activity as it stimulates our brain to become aware of conversations as well as activating our memory. That said, there are plenty of ways to socialize and get out there to interact with other people.

Things you might consider include:

· volunteering
· finding a hobby where you can socialize with other people
· taking a class like cooking, painting or exercising
· joining a community garden
· joining a book club, walking club or any social activity group that you might enjoy

The options are unlimited. If you live in a community or retirement residence, or have a friend who does, there are often events for residents to join in on. The next time you're walking down to the lobby or other social areas in the neighborhood, check out the calendar and see what's coming up!

Spiritual and Relaxation Activities

Taking care of our physical bodies is important but we also need to take care of our mental well-being, which needs to come from within. This means that you are tapping into spiritual and relaxation activities that will enhance a relaxed state, and decrease stress among other things.

Get Outside

One of the best things you can do to take care of your mental well-being holistically, is to get outside more. Even before the pandemic happened, many people found themselves spending a lot of time indoors, whether it was for work-related purposes or due to poor weather. However, on the days when the sun is shining and the temperature is lovely, you should spend some of your time outdoors, such as at a park, a public garden, or a public walking trail. It's a great way to improve your mental health, makes you feel less isolated, and can combat mental fatigue. Even sitting out on your porch or in your garden can do wonders, as long as you're getting fresh air and are connected to nature in some way.

Try Yoga

If the weather is poor, yoga is another excellent option to connect with yourself spiritually while finding a different way to get some gentle movement into your day. Yoga has plenty of benefits, including working on your breathing, strengthening your bones and muscles, and decreasing anxiety and stress. In addition, like Wall Pilates, you can adapt your yoga to use a chair for support. This option has become a favorite among seniors who are looking for ways to implement yoga into their lifestyle but are finding it hard to get into some of the poses.

Meditation

Meditation is an old practice that has been around for centuries, and is used to focus or clear inner clutter from your mind. There are plenty of ways to meditate, and depending on why you are meditating, it can help to calm your mind or decrease the symptoms of anxiety, depression, and stress. Meditating does not need to take a lot of time (5 to 10 minutes works best for most), but any of these can help you at a time when you need to unwind or calm a stressful mind:

- **Body scan:** In a body scan meditation, you'll take the time to use all of your senses to scan how your body is feeling. This meditation method is useful for those who have chronic pain which can cause you to lose focus or impact your sleep.

- **Mantra:** Mantra meditation uses the repetition of a phrase or sound in your head that you want to focus on.

- **Emotion-centered:** If you're dealing with a particular emotion, this method of meditation can help you focus on it.

- **Contemplation:** The contemplation method of meditation has you focus on a question or a contradiction without allowing your mind to wander. This is useful when you're trying to see a conflict from a different perspective.

- **Mindfulness:** Mindfulness meditation allows you to become more present in the moment and not let your mind wander to the past or what could happen in the future.

- **Movement:** Going for a walk in nature is a way to do a moving meditation. Some call this "Forest Bathing" if you're in a tree-like setting. That said, walking on the beach or through a park and letting the sights and sounds wash over you, is just as uplifting for the soul.

Practicing Gratitude

There are so many things we can be grateful for, but when we live in a busy world, we often forget to pause and reflect for a moment. This is where practicing gratitude comes into play.

Practicing gratitude is a habit that can boost your mental well-being. Like meditation, practicing gratitude doesn't need to take a lot of time. Some people like to write it down; however, you may even show your gratitude by checking in on your loved ones and being kind to others. However you decide to practice gratitude, when you make it a daily habit, you'll be surprised by how much your perspective will be a more optimistic one!

Journaling

Journaling is a valuable tool for all ages. It helps us organize our thoughts, brainstorm, plan our week, and keeps our brains active. Grab your wellness journal, and in the context of your holistic fitness journey, here's what journaling can do for you:

- **Reduces stress:** Stress has a significant impact on our health. It can weaken our immune system and increase symptoms of depression and anxiety. Regular journaling can help you manage your stress, work through frustrations, and help you see the bigger picture of what is going on in your life. By writing it all down, you can let the pent-up thoughts flow onto the paper, and away from your brain.

- **Boosts memory:** Journaling can help to recall dreams or fun memories, and practicing recall in general will help keep your brain sharp as a tack.

- **Enhances positive well-being:** Journaling can boost the creative part of your brain, allowing you to look at challenges with a creative perspective. The more you let your creativity flow, the more you'll have a more positive outlook overall.

- **Improves your relationships:** Journaling allows you to uncover parts of yourself. You can use these realizations to enhance and nurture your existing relationships.

There isn't a set way to journal because everyone does it differently. Some people like to journal to record anything and everything. Some want to write reflective journals to work through things that are currently happening or have happened in their lives. Some people journal to record what dreams they have in their hearts, and some want to make lists of goals. Some want to write about gratitude, but ultimately most people will end up doing a mix of any of these.

The bottom line is, you don't need anything fancy. Any way you journal will be relaxing and healthy for you, so just let things flow onto the pages and continue from there!

Taking Care of You

Taking care of yourself is holistic. It's about taking care of your mind by doing the things you love. It's about taking care of your body so that it has the right fitness, nutrients and hydration to continue functioning strongly, and lastly it means finding ways to take care of your emotional health. By incorporating these into your daily life, you can continue to build a fantastic, beautiful and vibrant life that's yours by your own design.

As Helen Mirren says:

> **"Your 40s are good. Your 50s are great. Your 60s are fab. And 70 is f*@king awesome!"**

I love the sound of such an awesome journey spanning decades up to and beyond 70, so use this book as a starting point, and keep designing your whole health from there!

CHAPTER 6:

OTHER RESOURCES BEYOND THE BOOK

Furthering Your Practice Online

You can find plenty of Wall Pilates routines online to enhance your Pilates practice. Some online tools, like YouTube videos, are free, while others have a subscription to access their content. Some of the paid subscriptions I have used, and I know many people who also enjoy these options, are:

· PilatesAnytime
· BetterMe

These two online resources give you an extensive library of various Pilates exercises. However, BetterMe tailors your Pilates routine to your needs, which is beneficial for having a routine that centers around your personal goals.

The above are two suggestions (to which I have no affiliation) but essentially, once you have the basics of Pilates down in a routine, there are many excellent online resources that can offer you a new challenge.

Connecting With Professionals

Beyond the comfort of your home, there is a whole world of Pilates to discover! If you can get to a studio, this is an excellent way to connect with a professional to enhance your Wall Pilates practice further. Finding a qualified instructor will help you:

· modify exercises to keep your body safe at all times.
· figure out which new Pilates exercises are good for you to do.

- to locate the correct muscles you should be using in the more advanced exercises.

Your next question may be how to know whether the instructor is qualified. The thing is, anyone can call themselves a Pilates instructor. However, a non-profit organization called the Pilates Method Alliance (PMA) can help consumers obtain the information they need about Pilates instructors.

In addition, look for studios or health clubs in your area and see if they share information on their instructor's background in Pilates. Connect with a physiotherapy clinic and see where they refer their clients to. No matter how you try to find an instructor, remember that Pilates is for every type of body, so finding an instructor that will work with your unique needs will deepen your practice, and help you move closer to your long-term goals.

No matter what you do at an outside studio, your continued Wall Pilates practice at home will keep you flexible and mobile in a quick and easy way that will enhance other activities that you seek.

Also, if you sign up for my VIP list, I'll send you helpful tips to keep you going, and I promise I won't overly spam you or try to upsell you. I only want to continue to support you and give you helpful ideas.

JOIN MY VIP LIST AND EARLY REVIEW TEAM!

Thank you for the time we've spent together - I truly appreciate it and hope that it's been a beneficial and worthwhile experience for you! Senior vitality is a passion of mine and I'm constantly striving to support a healthy, strong lifestyle for all ages! I have other books coming and would appreciate your early feedback as the books develop. By being a part of the early team, you'll receive free books and a say in the information I put out there! Also, reviews help others find the information they're seeking.

Please consider leaving a ★★★★★ review for this book using the QR code below, or if you have any questions, you can email me at:

<u>customercare@forever-fit-folks.com</u>

CONCLUSION

I hope you feel inspired and excited to add Wall Pilates into your daily life and reap all of the benefits.

Pilates is a beautiful practice. It's one of the safest and most accessible low-impact workouts for you, especially when you need to find workouts that are supportive and gentle on your body.

The basic routine is the first 28 days and then adding in the bonus and more advanced exercises makes up your second 28-day loop. Once you've completed both consistently, you'll be two months into your fitness routine and will have created a new healthy habit to take with you onto the next step towards total wellness.

I want to thank you for allowing this book to be a part of your wellness journey towards a better future. A lot of love has gone into this book, with the intent to help others. Your support and feedback are invaluable and if you enjoyed this book, please leave a review and help to give others a supportive way towards whole health!

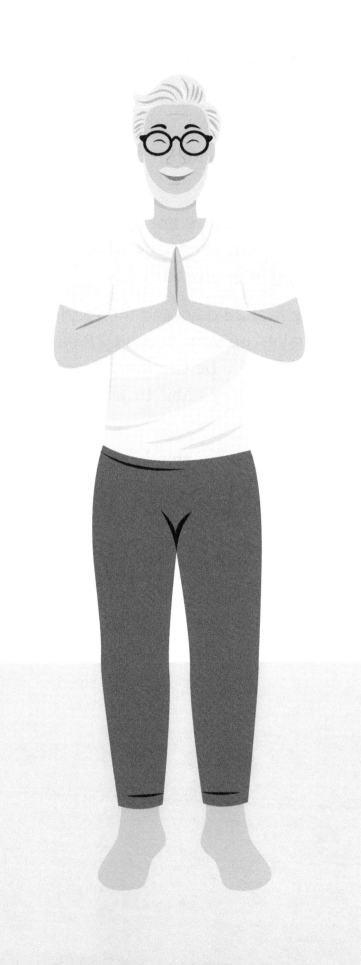

REFERENCES

Ackerman, C. (2018, July 5). *Positive mindset: How to develop a positive mental attitude.* PositivePsychology.com. https://positivepsychology. com/positive-mindset

Bandura, A. (2002). *Self efficacy in changing societies.* Cambridge University Press. https://books.google.ca/books?id=JbJnOAoLMNEC&printsec=frontcover&redir_esc=y#v=onepage&q&f=false

Berg, K. (2021). How to do a seated hip flexor stretch if you have Parkinson's [YouTube Video]. In *YouTube.* https://www.youtube.com/watch?v=O-Z-DKL86V_U&t=1s

Brain stimulating games and cognitive activities for older adults. (n.d.). The CareSide. https://www.thecareside.com.au/post/brain-stimulating-games-and-cognitive-activities-for-older-adults

Brown West-Rosenthal, L. (2022, May 17). *How a positive mindset can improve your workout.* The Output. https://www.onepeloton.com/ blog/how-a-positive-mindset-can-improve-your-workout

Brown, J. (2023, July 13). *Wall pilates for seniors: new effective and safe 21 exercises guide.* Fitt & Strong. https://fittandstrong.com/wall-pilates-for-seniors

Bucci, R. (2020, July 8). *The importance of warming up.* Results Physiotherapy. https://www.resultspt.com/blog/posts/the-importance-of-warming-up

Can breathing right during exercise help you avoid injury? (n.d.). OSR Physical Therapy. https://www.osrpt.com/2018/02/breathing-right-during-exercise

Cassata, C. (2019, September 20). *Why it's important to stay social as you age – and 5 ways to do it.* Healthline. https://www.healthline.com/health-news/staying-social-as-a-senior

centralhealthphysio. (2013). Seated roll down exercise [YouTube Video]. In *YouTube.* https://www.youtube.com/watch?v=LxQtAfz0PUo

Chalicha, E. (n.d.). *Chair pilates 101: all your questions answered.* BetterMe Blog. https://betterme.world/articles/chair-pilates

Chalicha, E. (n.d.). *The wall pilates app you need to switch up your at-home workouts.* BetterMe Blog. https://betterme.world/articles/wall-pilates-app

Chalicha, E. (n.d.). *Wall stretches: how to optimize your flexibility and mobility through wall stretching.* BetterMe. https://betterme.world/articles/wall-stretches

Cherry, K. (2023, February 27). *Self efficacy and why believing in yourself matters.* Verywell Mind. https://www.verywellmind.com/what-is-self-efficacy-2795954#toc-the-role-of-self-efficacy

Cordier, A. (2018, February 9). *5 reasons why warm up exercises are important.* Fit Athletic. https://fitathletic.com/5-reasons-warm-exercises-important

Digestive diseases statistics for the United States. (2014). National Institute of Diabetes and Digestive and Kidney Diseases. https://www.niddk.nih.gov/health-information/health-statistics/digestive-diseases

Eatough, E. (2023, May 8). *10 tips to set goals and achieve them.* BetterUp. https://www.betterup.com/blog/how-to-set-goals-and-achieve-them

Economou, E. (2023, September 15). *What is pilates breathing and why is it important?* Sixty and Me. https://sixtyandme.com/pilates-breathing

edvinas. (2023, July 13). *7 surprising wall Pilates benefits you need to know.* Wall Pilates. https://wallpilates.com/7-surprising-wall-pilates-benefits-you-need-to-know

edvinas. (2023, July 14). *Wall Pilates exercises for seniors.* Wall Pilates. https://wallpilates.com/wall-pilates-exercises-for-seniors

Elder Strength. (2022, June 10). *Lunges for seniors [the perfect leg strength exercise?].* https://elderstrength.com/lunges-for-seniors

Exercise of the week: seated arm circles. (2020, March 3). Courtney Medical Group. https://courtneymedicalgroupaz.com/2020/03/03/exercise-of-the-week-seated-arm-circles

Facts about falls. (2023, May 12). Centers for Disease Control and Prevention. https://www.cdc.gov/falls/facts.html

familydoctor.org. (2022, May). *Exercise and seniors* (D. S. Patel, Ed.). https://familydoctor.org/exercise-seniors

Finnie, D. (n.d.). *Wall pilates at home: the ultimate workout for a toned, tight and strong.* Pilates Moves You. https://pilatesmovesyou.com/wall-pilates-at-home-the-ultimate-workout-for-a-toned-tight-and-strong-core

14 examples of can do attitude. (n.d.). OpEx Managers. https://opexmanagers.com/examples-of-can-do-attitude

Forward leg swings | illustrated exercise guide. (n.d.). SPOTEBI. https://www.spotebi.com/exercise-guide/forward-leg-swings

George, A. (n.d.). *How to find a great pilates teacher.* Centerworks Online. https://centerworks.com/blogs/blog/find-a-pilates-teacher

Hamstring stretches: the anatomy of the hamstring. (n.d.). RedBox Fitness. https://www.redboxfitness.com/hamstring-stretches

High knees | illustrated exercise guide. (n.d.). SPOTEBI. https://www.spotebi.com/exercise-guide/high-knees

Hodge, J. (2021, June 12). *Return to exercise: 10 fitness journal prompts.* Hodge on Repeat. https://www.hodgeonrepeat.com/return-to-exercise-journal-prompts

Hong, A. R., & Kim, S. W. (2018). Effects of resistance exercise on bone health. *Endocrinology and Metabolism, 33*(4), 435. https://doi.org/10.3803/enm.2018.33.4.435

How and why to develop a growth mindset (as an older adult). (n.d.). Second Wind Movement. https://secondwindmovement.com/develop-growth-mindset

How older adults can get started with exercise. (2020, April 3). National Institute on Aging. https://www.nia.nih.gov/health/how-older-adults-can-get-started-exercise#activity

How to do a pelvic tilt exercise: a hinge health guide. (2023, April 28). Hinge Health. https://www.hingehealth.com/resources/articles/pelvic-tilt

How to stay hydrated for better health. (2021, August 23). Ncoa. https://www.ncoa.org/article/how-to-stay-hydrated-for-better-health

Howard, V. (n.d.). *Vernon Howard quotes.* GoodReads. https://www.goodreads.com/quotes/424452-always-walk-through-life-as-if-you-have-something-new

Inverarity, L. (2020, October 22). *How to do wall slides.* Verywell Fit. https://www.verywellfit.com/wall-slides-an-effective-quad-strengthening-exercise-2696607

Isacowitz, R., & Clippinger, K. (n.d.). *Learn three ways to control breathing during Pilates.* Human Kinetics. https://us.humankinetics.com/blogs/excerpt/learn-three-ways-to-control-breathing-during-pilates

Jones, R. (2023, February 23). *63 comfort zone quotes to push your personal boundaries.* Happier Human. https://www.happierhuman.com/comfort-zone-quotes-rj1

Journaling for seniors: how it enhances your brain health. (n.d.). Senior Helpers. https://www.seniorhelpers.com/ca/san-mateo/resources/blogs/journaling-for-seniors-how-it-enhances-your-brain-health

Kamau, C. (n.d.). *Wall angel exercise guide: techniques, benefits & muscles worked*. BetterMe. https://betterme.world/articles/wall-angel-exercise

Kamau, C. (n.d.). *Wall pilates equipment: Everything you need to know*. BetterMe. https://betterme.world/articles/wall-pilates-equipment

Kostaras, S. (2020, August 28). *How to do chair squats like a pro, even if you're a beginner*. Greatist. https://greatist.com/fitness/chair-squats

Kuzma, C. (2023, January 17). The best warm-up is a dynamic warm-up. *The New York Times*. https://www.nytimes.com/2023/01/05/well/move/dynamic-warm-up-exercises.html

Labonte, A. (2022, December 30). *Getting smart about goal setting for seniors*. HebrewSeniorLife. https://www.hebrewseniorlife.org/blog/getting-smart-about-goal-setting-seniors

Leonard, J. (2023, May 23). *What is learned helplessness*. MedicalNewsToday. https://www.medicalnewstoday.com/articles/325355

Mae, E. (2023, June 20). *10 fitness journal prompts to help you reach your goals*. ColoringFolder. https://coloringfolder.com/fitness-journal-prompts

Manheim, A. (2020, July 21). *Pilates lingo*. Pilates Anytime. https://www.pilatesanytime.com/blog/beginners/pilates-lingo

Martin, M. (2016, February 27). *Squats with ball against wall*. MelioGuide. https://melioguide.com/osteoporosis-exercises/wall-ball-squats-stability-ball

Marturana Winderl, A. (2022, January 11). *The 18 best exercises for knee pain, according to a physical therapist*. LIVESTRONG.COM. https://www.livestrong.com/article/13719074-exercises-for-knee-pain

Maxwell, J. C. (2000). *Failing forward: how to make the most of your mistakes*. Thomas Nelson Publishers.

Meditation. (2022, May 22). Cleveland Clinic. https://my.clevelandclinic.org/health/articles/17906-meditation

Melone, L. (n.d.). *7 dynamic warm ups.* Arthritis Foundation. https://www.arthritis.org/health-wellness/healthy-living/physical-activity/other-activities/7-dynamic-warm-ups

Menezes, L. (2020, August 24). *What is the mind-body connection?* Florida Medical Clinic. https://www.floridamedicalclinic.com/blog/what-is-the-mind-body-connection

Mind Tools Content Team. (n.d.). *Visualization* . MindTools. https://www.mindtools.com/a5ycdws/visualization

More Life Health Seniors. (2021). New seated warm up for seniors [YouTube Video]. In *YouTube.* https://youtu.be/MljaW8zv5bg?si=2h0-aTKR-wWv-dW7f

Mukhwana, J. (n.d.). *20 wall pilates benefits: you'll wish you knew about these sooner!* BetterMe. https://betterme.world/articles/wall-pilates-benefits

Munuhe, N. (n.d.). *What is wall Pilates? A guide for the beginner.* BetterMe. https://betterme.world/articles/what-is-wall-pilates

Musich, S., Wang, S. S., Kraemer, S., Hawkins, K., & Wicker, E. (2018). Purpose in life and positive health outcomes among older adults. *Population Health Management, 21*(2), 139–147. https://doi.org/10.1089/pop.2017.0063

Neck rolls | illustrated exercise guide. (n.d.). SPOTEBI. https://www.spotebi.com/exercise-guide/neck-rolls

Ogle, M. (2020, October 6). *How to do lateral breathing in Pilates.* Verywell Fit. https://www.verywellfit.com/learn-lateral-breathing-2704659

Ogle, M. (2020, November 5). *Create your own pilates workout routine.* Verywell Fit. https://www.verywellfit.com/create-your-own-exercise-program-2704649

Ogle, M. (2020, November 5). *How to do a wall roll down in Pilates.* Verywell Fit. https://www.verywellfit.com/standing-pilates-wall-roll-down-2704712

Ogle, M. (2021, May 21). *The 6 essential principles of Pilates*. Verywell Fit. https://www.verywellfit.com/six-pilates-principles-2704854

Older adults. (2023, April 16). Centers for Disease Control and Prevention. https://www.cdc.gov/physicalactivity/basics/older_adults/index.htm

Pack Health. (2018). Chair exercises: leg circles [YouTube Video]. In *YouTube*. https://www.youtube.com/watch?v=SPhvCLvINBQ

Parker, M. (2016, May 4). *13 of Audrey Hepburn's most inspiring quotes*. Time. https://time.com/4316700/audrey-hepburn-inspiring-quotes

Pereira, M. J., Mendes, R., Mendes, R. S., Martins, F., Gomes, R., Gama, J., Dias, G., & Castro, M. A. (2022). Benefits of pilates in the elderly population: a systematic review and meta-analysis. *European Journal of Investigation in Health, Psychology and Education, 12*(3), 236–268. https://doi.org/10.3390/ejihpe12030018

Perera, A. (2023, February 26). *The pygmalion effect: definition & examples*. SimplySociology. https://simplysociology.com/pygmalion-effect.html#How-the-Pygmalion-Effect-works

Pilates for upper back pain? 9 effective stretches for upper back pain. (n.d.). Complete Pilates. https://complete-pilates.co.uk/stretches-for-upper-back-pain

Pizer, A. (2022, September 29). *How to do a pelvic tilt*. Verywell Fit. https://www.verywellfit.com/how-to-do-pelvic-tilts-3566908

PMadmin. (2020, May 23). *Busting the myths about seniors and exercise*. Positive Maturity. https://www.positivematurity.org/busting-the-myths-about-seniors-and-exercise

Prendergast, C. (2023, September 17). *Exercise warmup for seniors*. Physio Ed. https://physioed.com/exercise-warmup-for-seniors

Prevention Magazine. (2013). Pilates on the wall: side leg lift [YouTube Video]. In *YouTube*. https://www.youtube.com/watch?v=vohhT9RvXaw

Purdie, J. (2022, October 26). *What is a cooldown?* Verywell Fit. https://www.verywellfit.com/what-is-a-cool-down-3495457

Quinn, E. (2022, March 11). *How to do a single-leg squat: proper form, variations, and common mistakes.* Verywell Fit. https://www.verywellfit.com/build-balance-and-strength-with-single-leg-squats-3119147#toc-other-variations-of-single-leg-squats

Ramos, T. (2023, August 18). *Squat with heel raise exercise guide: benefits, alternatives, and variations.* Generation Iron Fitness Network. https://generationiron.com/squat-with-heel-raise-exercise-guide

Relojo-Howell, D. (2021, June 25). *Understanding the connection between mind and body.* Psychreg. https://www.psychreg.org/connection-mind-body

Ryder, B. (n.d.). *When to breathe in pilates.* Pilates Secrets. https://pilatesecrets.com/when-to-breathe-in-pilates

Seated chair march. (n.d.). Falkirk Health and Social Care Partnership. https://livingwellfalkirk.lifecurve.uk/assess/areas-of-help/area/Bedroom/150ef1f9-4d5b-425c-91ef-02171349f1e4/groups/1b1542d3-95a0-4c36-9b97-fc2577c208d2/view/seated-chair-march

Sherrell, Z. (2023, May 26). *13 chair exercises that work your whole body.* Greatist. https://greatist.com/fitness/chair-exercises

6 leg lift exercises to strengthen your core. (2022, July 11). Cleveland Clinic. https://health.clevelandclinic.org/how-to-do-leg-lifts

6 tips for exercising safely as an older adult. (2021, December 15). LCMC Health. https://www.lcmchealth.org/touro/blog/2021/december/6-tips-for-exercising-safely-as-an-older-adult

Smith, J. (2020, September 25). *Growth vs fixed mindset: how what you think affects what you achieve.* Mindset Health. https://www.mindsethealth.com/matter/growth-vs-fixed-mindset

Smith, Z. (2018, April 6). *Ten best brain-stimulating activities for elderly loved ones.* Elder. https://www.elder.org/care-guides/24-hours-of-care-at-home/best-brain-stimulating-activities-elderly

Soniya. (2022, May 19). *How to do wall slides: tips, technique, correct form, benefits and common mistakes.* Sportskeeda. https://www.sportskeeda.com/health-and-fitness/how-do-wall-slides-tips-technique-benefits-more

Stefanacci, R. (2022, September). *Changes in the body with aging.* Merck Manuals Consumer Version; Merck Manuals. https://www.merckmanuals.com/en-ca/home/older-people%E2%80%99s-health-issues/the-aging-body/changes-in-the-body-with-aging

Taylor, J. L. (2009). *Proprioception* (L. R. Squire, Ed.). ScienceDirect; Academic Press. https://www.sciencedirect.com/science/article/abs/pii/B9780080450469019070

The 6 principles of Pilates. (n.d.). Fitness Advisory. Retrieved September 15, 2023, from https://www.fitnessadvisory.org/articles/the-6-principles-of-pilates

The importance of good blood circulation. (2023, March 23). Sanguina. https://sanguina.com/blogs/all/the-importance-of-good-blood-circulation

The origins of Pilates. (n.d.). Balanced Body. https://www.pilates.com/origins-of-pilates

Tight back? This simple seated side reach will help. (2021, December 6). Soul Central Pilates. https://www.soulcentralpilates.com/blog/pilates-seated-side-stretch-exercise

Valdez, E. (2021, August 4). *How to create the perfect home workout space.* UPPPER Gear. https://ca.uppper.com/blogs/news/creating-the-perfect-home-workout-space?shpxid=0bbd2b04-bc7d-442b-a8e8-02e-92411ac60

Velasco, M. (2021, August 21). *What is spine twist in pilates? How to, tips and modifications!* UMoveSg. https://umovesg.com/blogs/pilates-articles/what-is-spine-twist-in-pilates-how-to-tips-and-modifications

Wall sits with heel ups. (n.d.). Skimble. https://www.skimble.com/exercises/1090-wall-sits-with-heel-ups-how-to-do-exercise

Wallace, B. (2022, September). *Arthritis and joint pain.* University of Michigan National Poll on Healthy Aging. https://dx.doi.org/10.7302/6410

Warm-up and cool-down. (2022, December 1). NHS Inform. https://www.nhsinform.scot/healthy-living/keeping-active/before-and-after-exercise/warm-up-and-cool-down

Wenndt, L. (2022, October 5). *The 9 more chair exercises for seniors.* GoodRx Health. https://www.goodrx.com/well-being/movement-exercise/20-chair-exercises-for-seniors

What is a can-do attitude and how can you develop one? (2021, November 8). Twinkl. https://www.twinkl.com.ph/blog/what-is-a-can-do-attitude-and-how-can-you-develop-one

What is bone? (2023, May). National Institute of Arthritis and Musculoskeletal and Skin Diseases. https://www.niams.nih.gov/health-topics/what-bone

Why do the McConnell squat exercise? (n.d.). Complete Pilates. https://complete-pilates.co.uk/why-do-the-mcconnell-squat-exercise

Why gratitude works for senior health. (n.d.). Ethos. https://www.ethoscare.org/news/the-benefits-of-gratitude-in-older-adults

Why it's still important for seniors to set goals. (2021, January 11). CarePatrol. https://www.carepatrol.com/resources/blog/Why-Its-Still-Important-for-Seniors-to-Set-Goals_AE338.html

Wrist circles | illustrated exercise guide. (n.d.). SPOTEBI. https://www.spotebi.com/exercise-guide/wrist-circles

youmoveme. (2023, May 25). *Setting up the perfect home workout space.* https://youmoveme.com/blog/setting-up-the-perfect-home-workout-space

ZindzyGracia. (n.d.). *5 plank wall exercises for a powerful core.* BetterMe. https://betterme.world/articles/5-plank-wall-exercise

ZindzyGracia. (n.d.). *A beginner's guide to wall pushups: learn the basics of this effective exercise.* BetterMe. https://betterme.world/articles/wall-pushups

ZindzyGracia. (n.d.). *The beginner's wall plank guide for toned abs.* BetterMe. https://betterme.world/articles/wall-plank

ZindzyGracia. (n.d.). *Wall slides: a step-by-step guide to tone your core and upper body muscles.* BetterMe. https://betterme.world/articles/wall-slides

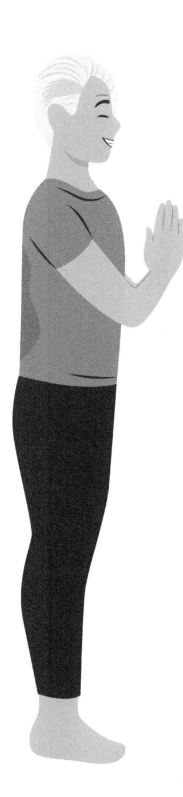

Made in the USA
Middletown, DE
14 March 2025

72654459R00122